MAKING THE MOST OF A NURSING FACILITY STAY

What to Expect for Your Loved One

Christine Ebrahim

Copyright © 2021 by Christine Ebrahim

All rights reserved. No part of this book may be reproduced or used in any manner without written permission of the copyright owner except for the use of quotations in a book review. For more information, address: christinelebrahim@gmail.com

FIRST EDITION

ACKNOWLEDGMENTS

This guide would not be possible without the expertise and input of other therapists and dedicated professionals working in nursing facilities, as well as friends and family. It is safe to say that one person doesn't know everything, and that person certainly isn't me! Therefore, I give my utmost thanks to the following individuals for dedicating their time to help in ways both big and small:

Thanks to Kris and Geoffrey Giron for their input early on and for providing me the feedback I needed to take those first steps. Thanks to the following therapists who edited, provided content ideas, and encouraged me: James Hu, OTR/L, Brianna Giruzzi, OTR/L, Juanita Verma, MOT, OT/L, CAPS, Amy Eiden, OTR/L, Kaylee Carino, MS, OTR/L, Irene Leung Bernardo, OT/L, Adriunna Boyd, MS, CCC-SLP, and Richa Singh, PT, MHA.

Thank you for the support and advice, John and Mark Ebrahim, Lance Abendan, and Denise Jones-Kazan. And of course, thank you to the members of the Facebook Geriatric OT, PT, and SLP Collaborative Group for giving me ideas of topics to be addressed in this guide.

TABLE OF CONTENTS

About the Author and Intent of Guide 8

Introduction 10
Who is this guide for? 11
How is this guide formatted? 11

Part 1: The Admission Process and Chain of Command 14
Why does the medical team recommend a nursing facility for my loved one? 15
How can I help with selecting a facility for my loved one? 15
What questions can I ask a potential facility? 17
What happens when my loved one first arrives at a nursing facility? 20
Who is paying for my loved one to be able to stay at a nursing facility? ... 22
Who should the facility contact if something is needed for my loved one? 24
What are some things that I should request to be contacted for? 25
What are everyone's roles and who do I speak to about different concerns? 25

Part 2: Belongings and Personal Care 34
Make Sure Everything is Labeled 35
How do I keep an inventory of my loved one's belongings? 36
How can I avoid my loved one's belongings becoming misplaced? . 36
What happens if my loved one's belongings go missing? 37
What toiletries should I bring my loved one from home? 38
Are there ways for my loved ones to get haircuts and other grooming services? 40
How often will my loved one be able to shower? 40
How is bathroom business conducted at nursing facilities? 41

Can anything be done if my loved one is having issues with continence?..42
Summary of Toiletries and Essentials from Home 44
What sort of clothing and shoes should I provide my loved one? How many pairs?. 45
What are some other items I could bring my loved one if they're staying long-term?. 46

Part 3: Mental and Physical Well-Being 48

How do I ensure my loved one stays engaged in the nursing facility?. 49
What are some ways I can encourage the memory and orientation of my loved one?. 50
How can I personalize my loved one's space to make them feel more at ease? 51
What can I do if my loved one is dissatisfied with their roommate(s)?. . . . 52
Should I bring anything to encourage my loved one's mobility?. 53
What can I do for my loved one if they are staying in bed too much? 54
How can I prevent my loved one from acquiring a pressure sore? 56
Why doesn't my loved one have bed rails? 57
What can be done to prevent my loved one from having falls?. 58
What sort of mental health services are available for my loved one?. 61
Does my loved one have access to an optometrist and vision services? 62
Does my loved one have access to dental care? How can they maintain their oral health? 62
My loved one sees a podiatrist. Will they have access to one in the facility? 63
Why is my loved one only given a certain texture of food? Why is their water thickened?. 63
What is aspiration and aspiration pneumonia? Why should I know about it? 64
How does my loved one leave the facility for appointments or other needs? 65
Even though my loved one lives in the facility, can they leave for visits?. . . 67

Part 4: Rehabilitation and Discharge Planning 70
Short-term Stays 71
How does rehabilitation assist my loved one to return home? 71
What can I do to prepare for my loved one that is returning home? 72
What should I do if my loved one needs more assistance than I can provide? 74
What options are available if my loved one isn't able to safely return home? 75
Long-term Stays 76
Why isn't my loved one on rehab anymore? When will they see a therapist again? 76
How do I ensure my loved one maintains their abilities when they are not on therapy? 79

Part 5: Advocacy and the Complaint Process 82
What rights does my loved one have while staying in a nursing facility? . . 83
How are nursing homes monitored for the care they provide? 84
How can I check in on my loved one's care? 85
How often should I visit my loved one? 86
What if visiting isn't an option? How else can I check in? 88
What are some signs to look for to ensure my loved one is receiving proper care? 90
What happens if my loved one's needs aren't being met or I need to make a complaint? 93
Who do I complain to within a facility if something goes wrong? 93
Who do I complain to outside of a facility about my loved one's care? What is a Long-Term Care Ombudsman? 94
Is there another avenue to file serious complaints? 95
What if I feel nothing has been done to address my concerns by any of these resources? 95

What are the different types of elder abuse?........................96
What are some warning signs of elder abuse?......................98
Who do I contact if I suspect my loved one's been abused?............99
What can I do if there is a change in my loved one's condition, health, or well-being? 100
What is a "NOMNC"? What if I don't agree with my loved one's insurance terminating coverage for staying at a SNF? 103

A Note On Covid-19 106

Conclusion..108

Checklist 112

Resources...116

References 126

ABOUT THE AUTHOR AND INTENT OF GUIDE

My name is Christine Ebrahim and I am an occupational therapist working in the sunny state of California. While I have only been in the skilled nursing environment for five years, I have found myself closely interacting with all sorts of individuals across all walks of life, and I am lucky to say I have learned a lot from them.

As an occupational therapist, I have the unique perspective of walking into a room and aiming to help an individual regain their independence, function, and—hopefully—their quality of life. Being an occupational therapist means recognizing what activities a person wants or needs to complete and finding the best ways to help them do that.

Core to occupational therapy's values is the belief that there are many ways to adapt and compensate for problems. A person who is now paralyzed from the neck down may need adaptive technology to allow them to navigate their world in a power wheelchair. An individual who had a hand injury may need to learn a new way to feed themselves.

We are always seeking ways to solve a wide range of issues, regardless of why an individual is struggling with them. We recognize that helping someone regain independence involves not only the physical factors but also the emotional and psychological ones. We need to cater to a person's comfort, well-being, and happiness before we can ever expect to effect change within their lives.

Many individuals I provide care for haven't stayed in a skilled nursing facility before. They don't understand a lot of aspects of their care. They—and their loved ones— have rightful concerns. From how long they can expect to be there, to what belongings they should bring, to who they can ask for help: their questions are understandable. Any one of us undergoing a transition would wonder the same things when finding ourselves in a new place.

In answering questions for patients and their loved ones, I have gathered a sense of the areas of concern most individuals have during their stay. Sometimes, it is as simple as directing a person to the right professional who can help. That alone can empower someone who otherwise feels lost or stressed.

It has become a passion of mine to be able to bring a resident or their family member comfort in knowing about their care. For this reason, I was inspired to share the knowledge I have with a wider audience, so I can provide some answers to anyone looking for them.

It is my goal to help as many residents of nursing facilities and their families feel confident in understanding their care. While this guide may not be comprehensive or provide all the answers, I have done my best to create this resource. I hope its intent remains clear: I want you to feel educated and empowered in navigating your loved one's nursing facility stay. Or, if it's you who's in a nursing facility, I hope you can begin to feel equipped with the knowledge to be your own self-advocate!

INTRODUCTION

Whether your loved one's stay in a skilled nursing facility is meant for short-term rehabilitation or long-term placement, the key to ensuring a positive stay is enriching yourself with the knowledge to best be involved and proactive.

Skilled nursing facilities (referred to sometimes as a nursing facility, nursing home, or SNF for short) are designed for individuals who need around-the-clock nursing care and for those who are not well enough to return home for one reason or another. The Center for Disease Control and Prevention (CDC) tells us that, in 2016, there were over fifteen thousand nursing facilities in the United States alone. In 2021, that number has probably increased!

Being such a large provider of care, some of us may know a relative or friend who's stayed in a SNF, but we may not have much knowledge beyond that. We aren't sure how a nursing facility operates to serve our loved one's needs. We want to become informed on how we may provide the best support or be involved in their care.

The good news is that learning about what to expect can empower you and your loved one in this journey. This guide will introduce you to answers to common questions I have heard asked both by patients and their family members alike.

Knowledge is power, as they say. Knowing what to expect from a nursing facility can provide you and your loved one the tools to make a SNF stay as productive as possible. Learning to navigate care within a SNF is paramount to ensuring a comfortable stay.

I hope that this guide will offer you a starting point in feeling empowered, enriched, and educated in your loved one's care. While I speak from the point of view of a therapist, I have done my best to provide the most comprehensive answers for some of the questions you may have.

Remember: the most accurate and specific answers will come from the professionals and organizations listed here; however, after reading, I hope that you will know a little more about how to navigate care within a SNF, tips for making a stay comfortable, as well as where to address some of your biggest questions and concerns.

Who is this guide for?

As the title implies, this guide was written and formatted to address families and friends of someone staying in a SNF. This format was selected to cover a more comprehensive set of topics that also speak to the areas a loved one would want to know about. Many individuals find themselves advocating for their loved ones from the outside with little direction or guidance.

You may be reading this as someone staying in a SNF yourself. You may also find that many answers relate to you individually. This guide is equally addressed to you, and hopefully, you find information that will help you on your journey of becoming your own advocate! I truly hope that you can make the most out of your nursing facility stay.

How is this guide formatted?

When browsing the table of contents, you may notice that this guide is divided into five parts, each addressing overarching topics. The guide is designed to be in a Q & A format to allow you to skip to questions that you may want answered. It can also serve as reading material from cover-to-cover. If you are just recently admitted into a nursing home or have a family member who is, reading it this way could also be beneficial.

It is important to note that a skilled nursing facility stay will vary based on whether your loved one's stay is planned for short-term (for recovery with a plan to return home) or if they are planning to take residence and live in a SNF for the long-term.

Parts 1, 2, 4 and 5 of this guide can be applied both to a long-term or short-term stay in a nursing facility. You may notice that Part 3 is most suited to address questions of long-term stays but some areas may also still apply to those staying short-term. Since a lot of information can overlap between short-term and long-term stays—they can encounter some of the same questions or issues— I have divided sections into short-term and long-term only when felt truly needed.

While some portions of this guide may not be relevant to your particular scenario, I hope that you can isolate the important parts to guide you on this journey.

PART ONE

The Admission Process and Chain of Command

Why does the medical team recommend a nursing facility for my loved one?

Most admissions into a skilled nursing facility (SNF) come from the hospital when an individual isn't safe to return home yet, does not have adequate care available, or is too medically complex to be managed without 24-hour nursing services.

While your loved one is hospitalized, they will be assessed for the safest place to go when they leave. If the team believes your loved one has ongoing medical or therapy needs, they may recommend a SNF as an option. An example of a medical need could be unmanaged pain, while an example of a therapy need could be trouble walking.

The team may also suggest a SNF if your loved one may not be safe to return directly home with the current level of help available there.

The team will explain their reasoning as to why they believe a nursing facility is the safest place to go after leaving the hospital. Of course, deciding to discharge to a SNF remains up to your loved one (or a designated person if they are not able to communicate their wishes). If your loved one decides upon a nursing facility, the hospital staff will provide options of SNFs that have openings in the preferred locations.

How can I help with selecting a facility for my loved one?

My recommendation would be to select a facility that is close in proximity to you or your family. Having your loved one stay at a facility within a reasonable distance from their support system can mean more frequent check-ins and an easier time coming by on short notice. Generally, having your loved one closer makes being involved a lot more manageable.

Understandably, families want to know a facility's reputation when sifting through options. One way to learn about a potential facility is to listen to firsthand accounts from family or friends that have stayed there or had a relative who did. It's better to pay attention to personal experiences over reviews, as reviews left on the internet could mainly be written by those who encountered issues. While reviews can certainly be helpful, they might not be representative of everyone's experiences.

Another way to gauge a facility's reputation is to look up where they lie on Medicare's Five-Star Quality Rating System. This is Medicare's system of rating nursing facilities on a scale of 1 to 5. The better a facility is considered, the higher the stars. Medicare looks at data from health inspections, the facility's staffing, as well as various quality measures when designating stars to a facility. You can compare nursing home ratings on Medicare's comparison site at www.medicare.gov/care-compare/.

I highly recommend touring potential facilities to gather a sense of what a stay may be like. Look at any residents you see. Do they appear active and busy, involved in a task? Or are they unoccupied, perhaps looking for something to do? Are there many call lights ringing? Are most residents in bed, or are they sitting up in chairs? These little glimpses can give you some information about a place.

What questions can I ask a potential facility?

Without any background knowledge, note that some of these questions may not make much sense to you at this time. That is absolutely okay. Before asking a facility questions, it may help to read about the different staff members who work within a SNF. You can read about that later in this section.

How long has the administrator been working there? The director of nursing? Rehabilitation staff?

Generally speaking, high staff turnover can be a sign of potential problems. An administrator and/or director of nursing who's remained consistent at a facility is a good sign that there is some sort of consistent leadership in place. Meanwhile, consistent rehab staff can indicate a strong team presence that can work well together to rehabilitate your loved one.

What is the ratio of nurses to residents? Certified nursing assistants (CNAs) to residents?

Since adequate staffing is vital in providing quality care, it is helpful to know how many nurses and CNAs are available per shift when looking for a facility. You can compare these numbers across options. Unfortunately, some facilities deal with staffing shortages; you may find this important to ask about.

Licensed vocational or practical nurses (LVNs or LPNs) can provide your loved one medication and communicate medical concerns with registered nurses (RNs) and doctors. In contrast, CNAs provide care with daily tasks (i.e., helping with dressing and bathing, bringing meals).

A recent study suggests that the ideal resident-to-CNA ratio is between 5 to 7 residents to 1 CNA for day and evening shifts and 11 to 12 residents to 1 CNA for night shifts. This means that a CNA should only handle care for that maximum number of residents at one time. In the same study, ratios for licensed vocational nurses (LVNs) vary greatly depending on how serious the cases were in the patients under their care. It ranged from 14 to 18 residents to 1 nurse for those needing extensive services to 24 to 28 in those patients needing less care. These ratios were for morning and evening shifts. Night shifts, in general, seem to require a little less nursing staff care (Harrington, Dellefield, Halifax, Fleming, & Bakerjian, 2020).

These numbers are only suggestions. The actual ratios can vary greatly depending on a lot of factors, like the type of patients a facility serves and how serious their individual needs are. Several states have minimum requirements for staffing facilities, and there are also federal laws around nursing home staffing. Some argue, however, that these minimum standards are not sufficient for providing proper care. Therefore, I would recommend comparing staffing across potential facilities for your loved one.

How often do the doctors at this facility come to assess residents?

Most medical assessments in SNFs occur by nurses and are relayed to doctors, who receive these updates and act accordingly. These doctors and their team of nurse practitioners and/or physician assistants also assess the residents who are under their care. It would be helpful to know approximately how often these visits occur at a potential facility.

What are your visiting hours and how am I allowed to visit safely?

In an ever-evolving public health climate, it is important to establish how you may visit your loved one once they are in the facility and what these visiting hours consist of. Knowing this in advance can ease both your loved one's mind as well as your own as they make this transition.

Do you have a designated area for your residents to spend time outdoors?

It is beneficial to the health and well-being of everyone to be able to go outside and get some fresh air. It would help to ask about whether your loved one will have access to a safe and comfortable outdoor space at their potential facility.

Does this facility have a restorative nursing program in place?

This is an especially important question if there's a chance your loved one's stay may be long-term. Restorative programs (discussed in greater depth later in this guide) are a way to ensure that your loved one maintains their functional abilities once they are no longer on physical, occupational, or speech therapy services. You want to make sure you select a facility that has this sort of program in place.

What sort of activities do you have in place for residents?

We all want to ensure our loved one has activities around them to keep them engaged. A facility with a healthy activities department will likely include games, movies, crafts, and various other entertainment to provide leisure for your loved one.

Will my loved one be able to visit home?

If your loved one plans to stay in a facility for long-term care, it would be helpful to know current options for visiting home and how this is safely arranged. In my experience, an individual staying in a nursing facility really values the opportunity to take outings to spend time with family and friends.

These are just some of the few questions you may want to ask, but you also may have questions of your own that are important to you or your loved one. I suggest writing them down before making phone calls or visits!

What happens when my loved one first arrives at a nursing facility?

Once your loved one has decided on a facility, they will be transported there when the hospital doctor deems it safe. The hospital will send over all of the necessary information, such as medications and diagnoses, and there will be a report given from the hospital nurse to the admitting nurse at the facility. This conversation will cover all aspects of your loved one's care: from how oriented they are, to their preferences, and any concerns the staff should be immediately aware of.

If your loved one is having any pain, it might be helpful that they request pain medicine at the hospital prior to heading over to the facility in case there are any delays in their medications transferring over. To avoid any potential issues, make sure your loved one is comfortable and prepared for the transition.

Upon admission, a *skin assessment* occurs, where a nurse may ask your loved one to turn side to side and closely inspect every part of the body to ensure no cuts, wounds, or pressure sores are present that they are not already aware of.

This process will be explained to your loved one so they know what to expect and may be repeated at a certain interval (daily, weekly, etc). Keep in mind that during this check—and during any care given, for that matter— your loved one is able to request for male- or female-specific staff. Some people are simply more comfortable with one or the other during these private moments, which is absolutely okay.

On the first day or two of admission, there is a lot of paperwork to be signed and interviews to be conducted. Most departments will need to go through their own assessments with your loved one and may reach out to you if you are a designated contact and your loved one isn't able to answer for themselves.

You may wonder how a facility becomes aware of what your loved one can or cannot do for themselves. Most of the time, physical and occupational therapists will conduct initial assessments and communicate your loved one's current level of function with the rest of the team so that everyone may assist them as much as possible within any limitations they have. A speech-language pathologist (SLP) will also relay information around safe diet textures, swallowing strategies, mental status, and/or ways to communicate with your loved one if they have issues in any of these areas.

Those first few days after your loved one's admission can be a rollercoaster of emotions. You may have many questions, and the answers may need to come from different individuals responsible for your loved one's care. I strongly recommend writing your questions down in a notebook and keeping a log of the answers you receive to ensure you don't need to recall everything from memory.

Care Conference Meetings

If you are a designated contact for your loved one, you may be called within the first few days about a care conference meeting. This is a meeting that happens upon admission to discuss all facets of your loved one's care. The meeting is usually attended by representatives from all departments, including nursing, social services, rehabilitation, dietary, and activities. You will be familiarized with these departments in an upcoming section.

This conference is an opportunity to ask anything you need to know about your loved one's care. The team will try to establish goals with you. It is a good idea to write down any questions you have to bring to this meeting, as well as any outcomes to track whether a follow-up will be necessary for the coming weeks.

If someone is present for your loved one in this conference that does not speak or understand English, be sure to request for a translator. You may also request a translator during any important communication throughout your loved one's stay.

Care conferences typically occur shortly after admission, at discharge, or quarterly if your loved one's stay is long-term. Ask your loved one's facility what their conference schedule typically looks like.

Who is paying for my loved one to be able to stay at a nursing facility?

A stay in a nursing facility can be more costly than an extravagant hotel. Considering around-the-clock nursing care and services, meals, rehabilitation, and more, the nightly stay in a nursing facility ranges in the hundreds, if paid out of pocket. Now factor in a month-long stay. This number can turn into upwards of seven to nine thousand!

Luckily, a person (sometimes referred to as a resident) admitted into a nursing facility usually has an insurance provider that pays for some or all of the cost of staying there initially. Sometimes, there is a share of cost that a resident is responsible for paying as well. This is an amount of the total cost of care that the insurance has designated the individual to pay.

If your loved one is planning for a short-term stay: Medicare Part A and HMO insurance providers will typically pay for the stay until they believe they can return home. Sometimes, HMO providers will discontinue coverage earlier than hoped and may require an appeal process to try and continue the stay uninterrupted.

With Medicare, the first 20 days are covered at 100%, days 21 through 100 requires a *share of cost* percentage to be paid, and after 100 days, the individual becomes responsible for *all* payments within that stay (U.S. Centers for Medicare & Medicaid Services, n.d.) If your loved one has secondary insurance or long-term care insurance that can help pay for costs, you can work with social services to supplement their coverage.

If your loved one is planning for long-term care: Medicare and HMOs do not pay for long-term care stays. They will only provide coverage for medical services that are rendered and not usually *custodial care* (care with daily living tasks, such as getting dressed or bathing).

It is in a situation such as this that having long-term care insurance comes in handy; however, if your loved one falls within a lower income bracket, each state has its own medical assistance program (such as MediCal in California and Medicaid for the Elderly and People with Disabilities in Texas) that can help with paying for some of the long-term custodial care costs. If you need help with this—or have any questions around the financial aspect of care— the facility's social services director(s) should be well-acquainted with the services available in your state and what options your loved one has financially for long-term care.

Who should the facility contact if something is needed for my loved one?

It is very important to note that information can only be given out to individuals on a resident's approved list due to the importance of protecting health information.

With this in mind, it may be best to designate a primary contact for your loved one's care. Often, when too many individuals want to be informed about care, different people may be contacted for different concerns. It can become quite confusing for both your family and the facility staff.

Having one or two individuals receive updates from the facility regarding care does place a lot of responsibility on those individuals. If you are the primary contact for your loved one, it will help to write down any information provided by staff in a log. Keeping a list of any questions/concerns that other family members have would assist with organization, too. This will allow you to have a physical record rather than trying to manage everything in your head.

Acting as a representative for an entire family can be a big responsibility. There is no harm in switching the role to somebody else if needed, or designating two people (who keep close contact with one another) to both be the contacts. The key is to keep your loved one's care a unified effort and avoid the confusion that comes with too many cooks in the kitchen.

What are some things that I should request to be contacted for?

In addition to case conferences and calls regarding discharge planning, you can also ask to be contacted for any medication changes that the doctor orders for your loved one. In addition, you may also request to be informed when medical appointments are made. If your loved one is receiving therapy services, you can request the rehab department to reach out to you in case of any issues with your loved one completing their therapy (i.e., your loved one is consistently refusing participation for one reason or another).

What are everyone's roles and who do I speak to about different concerns?

The chain of command in a SNF can be complicated to understand at first, but once you figure out who manages what, it will be easy to effectively track down the right person to speak with about your loved one's care.

Here are some of the roles within a nursing facility that you may want to familiarize yourself with:

Administrator

The administrator is the head of the facility. They oversee every department and handle the big picture issues rather than the day-to-day tasks, which are often delegated to department heads. Still, they are informed about what occurs within the SNF by their department heads and try to maintain involvement as much as possible.

Certified Nursing Assistant (CNA)

If there is one group of individuals to make sure you connect with, it's your loved one's CNAs. They are, by and far, the people who spend the most time with them. Depending on the amount of physical assistance your loved one needs, they provide any self-care needs, including bathing, toileting, dressing, and more. They also can take vitals and relay any concerns to the nurse. Often, your loved ones will first tell their CNA that they are having pain or an issue, who will then report that to the nurse.

Charge Nurse

The charge nurse or station nurse is the nurse (either a Registered Nurse or Licensed Vocational/Practical Nurse) assigned to your loved one's care on any given shift. The charge nurse provides medical interventions, such as giving medications, monitoring vitals, and calling the doctor for concerns. Keep in mind that an RN is able to perform some interventions that an LVN/LPN cannot, such as starting an IV for medication.

Typically, SNFs have three shifts: AM from around 7 am to 3 pm, PM from around 3 pm to 11 pm, and nocturnal (or noc) from around 11 pm to 7 am. The nurses and CNAs will typically rotate at these timeframes. Ideally, you'll have the same few CNAs and nurses treating your loved one, as they've gotten to know them and their needs over time. However, it is possible that your loved one won't always have consistent nursing staff, depending on the facility and their staffing.

Nurse Supervisor

The nursing supervisor directly supervises all of the charge nurses on any given shift. They are the people whom the nurses can turn to first if an issue comes up that they are uncertain how to handle. They can be a great contact for a wide range of nursing-related questions or concerns.

Wound Care Nurse

A wound nurse is a nurse who has specialized in the assessment and treatment of skin breakdown, most notably bedsores or pressure sores. If you have any skin-related concerns about your loved one, if your loved one has a wound, or if you are concerned about your loved one developing a wound, the wound care nurse is a great resource.

Director of Nursing (DON)

The DON oversees all nurses, wound nurses, and nurse supervisors of the facility. This individual may sometimes have an assistant, depending on the facility size. The DON can be a great resource if you have not been able to have your need addressed by the rest of the nursing staff or if your loved one's concerns are complex and require wide-scale intervention.

Nurse Practitioner (NP) and Physician Assistant (PA)

More often than not, a SNF doctor manages patients in more than one facility. Because of this high caseload, they often appoint NPs and PAs to handle the day-to-day medical care of residents in a nursing facility. NPs and PAs visit a facility regularly and have good knowledge of residents and their needs. Under the doctor's supervision, NPs and PAs can adjust medication doses, prescribe medications, order labs and tests, and handle most concerns around your loved one's medical care.

As they are also seeing patients in multiple facilities, it may be difficult to get a direct hold of your loved one's NP or PA. That is why speaking with the nurse, nurse supervisor, and/or the DON would be the most effective route in regards to medical concerns, as they can then contact the rest of the medical team on your behalf.

Facility Doctor

A medical doctor (M.D. or D.O.) is assigned to your loved one when they are admitted into the facility and is typically different from your loved one's usual primary care physician (PCP). During their stay, the assigned medical doctor functions as your loved one's PCP. If your loved one plans to discharge from the facility, they will then be transitioned back to the care of their original PCP.

The appointed physician oversee the entirety of your loved one's care but may not be regularly present in-person. A lot of what they know about your loved one is communicated to them by the nursing staff listed above, as well as the NPs and PAs. As mentioned, it is helpful to communicate with those staff members effectively and understand their important roles.

Case Manager

The case manager plays an important part in bridging all aspects of your loved one's care. In nursing facilities, case managers are most often also licensed nurses whose goal is making sure care is coordinated across all disciplines. They are also central to planning for a safe return home. Case managers are in contact with doctors, rehabilitation staff, nurses, and other members of the care team in an effort to organize your loved one's care effectively. They are great to turn to if you are unsure where to direct your questions, since they'll often know who may be the best person for you to speak with.

Director of Rehab (DOR)

The DOR is the manager of the rehabilitation department and is your point of contact for anything therapy-related. This individual is also a therapist themselves. Under this person's supervision are physical therapists, occupational therapists, and speech-language pathologists. It is beneficial to understand their distinctions so that if your loved one needs any of their services, you may better know what to request:

> ### *Physical Therapists (PTs) / Physical Therapy Assistants (PTAs)*
> PTs and PTAs work with all sorts of mobility-related issues, from being able to roll in bed, to standing and walking, to being able to manage stairs and sidewalks. They can decide what sort of mobility aid your loved one needs to be safe: be it a cane, walker, wheelchair, or something else. If your loved one is a long-term care resident, they may be able to step in when there has been a decline in your loved one's ability to get up from bed, walk, or in their overall strength, balance, coordination, and endurance. PTs/PTAs are also wonderful advocates and educators who can provide training to staff regarding the best ways to help your loved one up and moving safely.

Occupational Therapists (OTs) / Certified Occupational Therapy Assistants (COTAs)

OTs and COTAs are vital in the rehabilitation process and take different roles in different settings. In SNFs, OTs work mainly with dysfunctions in activities of daily living (ADLs), such as using the bathroom, dressing, feeding oneself, and showering. They will perform these activities with your loved one and assist them in regaining independence through different interventions. If your loved one needs to be able to prepare meals, clean, or do laundry, these tasks may also be addressed. OTs can work on the balance, coordination, cognition, and endurance necessary to perform daily activities. They can also educate nursing staff on how to assist an individual through these tasks safely. As there is so much within the scope of OT, I would encourage you to do further research on what they can do to help!

Speech-Language Pathologists (SLPs) / Speech-Language Pathology Assistants (SLPAs)

SLPs are critical in the care of a lot of individuals admitted into nursing facilities. SLPs handle not only issues of speech and language but are also specialists in cognition function, swallowing, and determining safe diet textures. A wide range of conditions can affect a person's ability to swallow safely, and an SLP must assess a person who has had a change in this function to determine what is best for them to be able to consume safely. SLPAs are less commonly found in the SNF environment but are certified to assist the SLP with implementing their chosen interventions. SLP interventions may include performing oral-motor exercises to improve swallow function, learning compensatory strategies to improve memory and orientation, and much, much more. Just as with OT, I would recommend doing further research on the many areas an SLP can address!

Restorative Aides / Restorative Nursing Assistants

These individuals (referred to as RNAs or RAs) are CNAs who have received specialized training in restoring and rehabilitating residents to maintain or achieve their maximum level of functioning. RNAs can assist patients through an exercise program, provide instructions to ensure someone is dressing on their own, or even ensure someone is following safe swallowing strategies. RNAs usually see patients who are not on therapy but can be involved while a patient is on therapy services as well. An RNA will typically follow a plan set forth by a PT, OT, or SLP. You can learn more about the important role of RNAs later in this guide.

Social Services Director

The social services director's many roles can include scheduling transportation, finding housing for those looking to discharge and are uncertain of location, helping with financial concerns, applying for supplemental insurance, handling complaints, and directing concerns to the proper departments. The social services director sometimes has an assistant working under them, given that their department manages a lot of things. Larger buildings may even have more than one director. These individuals are a wonderful resource and, like the case manager, can be seen as the jack-of-many-trades.

Activity Director

An activity director has the unique role of creating leisure for the residents at a facility. They are tasked with coming up with different activities, both social and individual, and learning about each resident's interests and hobbies in hopes of creating entertainment and recreation. Activity directors also typically have assistants that are providing the day-to-day leisure interventions. They are great to talk to if your loved one's stay is long-term (and also short-term) to ensure their leisure is prioritized. You can also reach out if you have questions about how your loved one can be more actively engaged in their day-to-day life in the facility.

Dietary Supervisor

The dietary supervisor oversees all of the dietary staff members preparing your loved one's meals. They are present to ensure that dietary restrictions, such as a fluid restriction or limited salt diets, are communicated to their staff and that food is being prepared according to the ordered diet. They are the person to speak to about specific requests for a loved one's meals, food preferences, and meal-related concerns.

Registered Dietician (RD)

A registered dietician keeps track of the specific nutritional needs of residents. Like medical doctors, they also typically manage a caseload over multiple SNFs. They can order supplemental nutrition or evaluate the effectiveness of a particular diet that is currently in place. They are involved, too, when weight loss is at play in an attempt to investigate how to assist with this.

Clinical Psychologist

Many facilities have a psychologist that makes visits between different facilities. They are usually referred to by the medical team and can also request that the individual see the psychiatrist for mental health concerns that involve potential medication needs. If you have concerns about your loved one's mental health, you can ask your loved one's nurse about what psychological services are available to them.

Maintenance Supervisor

The Maintenance Supervisor takes care of issues that arise in the environment and is vital to ensuring your loved one has fully functioning services in their rooms. They can assist with climate issues, fixing air conditioning or heating problems, a faulty TV, malfunctions with beds— virtually any room or equipment-related issues. They are a wonderful resource!

—

Knowing who manages what in a SNF can decrease the likelihood of being redirected from person to person when attempting to resolve a concern. To avoid this potential back and forth, it helps to know who to speak with before ever having an issue!

PART TWO

Belongings and Personal Care

Make Sure Everything is Labeled

If there is only one thing to remember regarding your loved one's belongings, it's that having everything labeled is absolutely necessary. Every single item that is handed to your loved one should be clearly labeled or labeled by the facility. This even includes items you might not even have considered labeling: books, denture containers, glasses cases, socks, shoes, and even sometimes snacks.

Imagine a dorm room or even a house with a lot of people living inside. Items tend to go missing. Now, remember that your loved one's stay in a nursing facility isn't unlike a dorm: several individuals can share a room, there are generally communal showers, and centralized services are available (meals, laundry, etc). Items are bound to become mixed up, not by fault of any one particular person, but by nature of the living environment.

Before labeling your loved one's belongings, make sure to check with their facility regarding their individual policy. Some facilities only accept items that they label themselves, while others request that you provide the labeling.

You can request to have your loved one's important items safely locked, such as purses, wallets, and money. Expensive or valuable items that are not used regularly, such as fine jewelry, are better kept home to ensure these don't get misplaced. [1]

Even with the best labeling and organization system in place, your loved one may still have something turn up missing from time to time. But to decrease

---

[1] Be mindful that weight loss can cause rings and bracelets that once fit to fall off. In addition, swelling can cause issues with jewelry becoming too tight. Consider both of these when determining what valuables to bring home.

the odds, making sure items are labeled will give them the best shot at keeping their belongings safe.

How do I keep an inventory of my loved one's belongings?

Now that we've established that items can be misplaced in SNFs, we can consider a method of keeping track of your loved one's belongings. While facilities keep inventories of a resident's belongings, it would be wise to also keep a personal list of the items you provide your loved one.

If possible, being present when the facility conducts its own inventory check (usually on the day of admission or when you provide a new item) would be ideal to ensure your list and their list are the same. If you're unable to be present, you can ask for a copy of their inventory. This way, if something turns up missing, you've already confirmed on their end that the item was present when your loved one arrived (since they also have it logged).

How can I avoid my loved one's belongings becoming misplaced?

Something I've seen help with keeping things where they belong is the use of storage caddies and organizational bins. Ideally, these bins are separated by category (i.e, toiletries bin, crafts bin). By far, I have noticed individuals who have a neat assignment of where their items go, or a system of organization, tend to experience less misplaced belongings.

Having bins for items of different categories will keep both staff and your loved one from constantly guessing the whereabouts of their essentials.

I had one particular resident feel empowered by her organization system. Although she was physically unable to reach for all of her belongings, she could describe its location to you perfectly (*"Please bring me my glasses, which are in the green cubby, third section to the left."*) I could tell she took great pride in knowing the whereabouts of her essentials and retained a sense of independence by organizing her place in a way she wanted.

Furthermore, if you have the ability to launder your loved one's clothing, it can greatly decrease the chance of their favorite clothing pieces going missing. Often, a loved one will set a bin in their loved one's closet and inform staff to deposit clothing there, rather than sending it to the laundry. Check with your loved one's facility around rules for washing your loved one's clothing if this is something you'd like to undertake.

What happens if my loved one's belongings go missing?

Loved ones may not realize the hard work laundry staff put into organizing clothes and returning them to their owners. In many cases, laundry makes every effort to find the owner of unlabeled items. Whether your loved one's items were simply unlabeled, fell victim to a fading label, or just misplaced, facilities have rules in place to compensate for lost items.

If something does end up missing, every facility has its own policy regarding how to handle this. It would be smart to familiarize yourself with it. At most facilities I have worked in, the social services department handled lost item concerns. Usually, there was some sort of reimbursement or consolation provided when those items could not be found.

Regular checks of your loved one's living area are a good way to ensure they are not going without their essentials and valuables. If your loved one isn't able to check their belongings for themselves and you are not able to be present, you can always ask their CNA to check for specific items and/or what may need to be restocked.

What toiletries should I bring my loved one from home?

If your Loved One's Stay is Short-Term

Bringing your loved one some comforts and familiar essentials from home, even if their stay is short-term, may help with the transition and make their overall nursing facility stay smoother.

The standard toiletries I've seen provided by nursing facilities are toothbrushes, toothpaste, denture cups, denture adhesive cream (sometimes), nail clippers, combs, deodorant, brushes, shampoo, body wash, lotion, shaving cream, and razors. Of course, these items vary from facility to facility and state by state. It would help to check with your loved one's facilities about what items are provided to them.

That being said, your loved one may be used to their tried and true brands and feel more comfortable using them. If that is the case, something as simple as making sure your loved one has their personal toothpaste and toothbrush would be a kind gesture.

Despite its importance, most facilities I have worked in do not carry floss in their inventory. As flossing is such a vital part of oral hygiene, providing your loved one with this simple item is one of the best things you can do to keep their oral health prioritized. [2]

---

[2] Check with your loved one's nursing staff around whether they are able to have floss brought to them, as some rules may affect doing so.

Furthermore, if your loved one has dentures, check whether their facility provides denture cleaning tablets to maintain oral hygiene.

Also, if your loved one has dentures, glasses, or hearing aids, bringing them in clearly marked and labeled containers will help keep their belongings organized. Families can also request to store these important items in the nurse's cart or locked in the medicine room.

Other items may be appreciated, depending on your loved one's preferences, such as shampoos and body washes, deodorant, razors—even chapstick. Nobody likes dealing with dry lips!

If your Loved One's Stay is Long-Term

You may want to consider bringing a little more in terms of comfort if your loved one plans to stay at a nursing facility for the long-term.

In addition to the standard toiletry supplies discussed above, you may want to consider other items that your loved one may have used regularly before their move into a nursing facility: a blow dryer, a table mirror, skincare products, and makeup. I had a resident once who wouldn't start her therapy without first putting her lipstick on!

Hearing aids and dentures should be clearly marked and labeled within designated containers. Ideally, extra batteries for hearing aids will ensure your loved one never has to go without them when a new set is needed or if a set goes missing. You may want to discuss with CNA staff how often the hearing aid batteries typically need to be replaced.

If your loved one has long hair, consider bringing a pack of hair ties, bobby pins, and clips. This is something I find myself supplying my residents when they do not receive them from family.

If there are essential aspects of care unique to your loved one, make sure it is added to your loved one's plan of care, so that there is documentation of what specific needs are being addressed (i.e., ensuring staff offer your loved one their hearing aids daily or providing headphones with music as a source of entertainment).

Are there ways for my loved ones to get haircuts and other grooming services?

Yes! Most nursing facilities hire beauticians that come on a scheduled basis. These beauticians can usually provide cutting, trimming, styling, and shaving services. Check with your loved one's facility to determine who is in charge of setting up these services and the costs associated with them.

How often will my loved one be able to shower?

Showers in most nursing facilities are on a rotating schedule. The frequency of how often a resident is assisted into the shower room varies from facility to facility, so you may want to ask your loved one's facility about their schedule (i.e., twice weekly, thrice-weekly). Your loved one will also generally be placed on either an AM or PM shower schedule, so if your loved one will most certainly refuse a shower in the morning, it is best that this is communicated with staff. Everyone has a preference for bathing time, and it is important to do our best to accommodate that.

Since showers are almost never daily, your loved one could benefit from their own supply of wet wipes. While facilities have these on hand, your loved one having their own wipes may make them feel more comfortable using as many as necessary. Keep in mind that your loved one will be able to clean themselves as needed between showers with either soapy washcloths or wet wipes—whichever they prefer. They will receive assistance from their CNA to do this if they are not able to on their own.

One thing to note is that different wings of your loved one's facility might follow different shower schedules. For example, your loved one may have a shower scheduled for Monday and Wednesday afternoons and then is transferred to another part of the facility on Wednesday morning. This new section may place him onto Tuesday and Friday showers. In a situation such as this, you may need to make sure that they receive their shower as previously planned. In addition, you may find that you need to communicate your loved one's preferred showers (mornings or afternoons) so that they can best work around their preferences.

There are unique instances where someone may not be able to shower for some time. For example, a resident who has recently undergone surgery and has not received orders from the doctor that they are safe to resume showering may need to stick to *sponge bathing* (use of wet, soapy washcloths to keep clean outside the shower). This may be due to healing a wound or incision or for another medical reason. You can ask your loved one's staff to keep in contact with you regarding when your loved one is safe to resume showering again.

How is bathroom business conducted at nursing facilities?

While it may not have been something you thought about before, staying informed about your loved one's toilet use may be very important now. As an occupational therapist, one of my main goals is making sure someone can use the bathroom as independently as possible. I have unfortunately witnessed some residents using diapers (or briefs) to relieve themselves when a visit to the bathroom could have been an option. This is not only a major issue of dignity; it can also encourage the development of incontinence.

The good news is that prioritizing toileting needs and creating a plan can prevent these sorts of problems from ever happening.

If your loved one is even partially continent (able to determine when they need to use the restroom), it is important that a toileting plan is established and followed. If your loved one is safe to mobilize to the bathroom without assistance, that is the easiest option as it doesn't require staff involvement; however, if mobility is a challenge, an occupational therapist can determine the safest way to get to a toilet.

There should always be a way. An individual who can't make it to the bathroom but can make it a few feet from their bed should be capable of using a bedside *commode* [3]. Even someone unable to get out of bed can use a *bedpan* [4] to ensure they are toileting with the contents removed immediately. Ask about these options, if needed.

Can anything be done if my loved one is having issues with continence?

If your loved one expresses new or worsening incontinence, it would be good to bring it up to the medical team for evaluation (i.e., your loved one's nurse who

---

3 a portable toilet
4 a receptacle used for toileting in bed

can relay it to the doctor). In addition to a medical assessment for underlying causes, there are other ways to encourage continence.

Whether someone is continent, partially incontinent, or fully incontinent, a toileting schedule is very useful. Toileting schedules are programs established to ensure regular bathroom visits happen. Regardless of an individual knowing when they need to go or not, having a toileting schedule can be beneficial to their health and well-being.

Toileting schedules can be determined by patterns observed by staff, or they can be timed (i.e., a bathroom visit every 3-4 hours). This encourages a person to regularly attempt to use the bathroom, even if they do not know when they need to go. Having your loved one on a regular toileting schedule will keep their skin clean, encourage bathroom use, and give them the chance to participate in a routine activity.

If your loved one qualifies for therapy, you can ask the occupational therapist about your desire to create a routine for them. The director of nursing (DON) can also be another option for inquiring about this sort of program. And remember: as personal as it can be, try to remain informed about how your loved one is going about their business. It's important!

Pull-Up Briefs

If your loved one can manage their clothing some or all of the time, pull-up briefs or incontinence underwear may be a good option to simplify the bathroom process. Many facilities use a style of brief that is attached at the front via sticky tabs. This makes changing briefs in beds easier for CNAs but presents a challenge for individuals if they are trying to manage their clothing on their own.

Pull-up briefs are not usually provided by facilities I have personally worked in. This style of brief is easier to manage when pulling them up and down. Be prepared to possibly supply your loved one with their own pull-ups if this is something they can use.

Summary of Toiletries and Essentials from Home

These are some items you should consider labeling and bringing from home to provide your loved one with the most comfort, especially if their stay is long-term:

- Toothbrush (electric or standard) and toothpaste
- Shampoo and conditioner
- Hairbrush or comb
- Blow dryer, if used
- Deodorant
- Floss
- Dentures and denture adhesive (if used)
- Denture cleaning tablets (if not provided)
- Lotion
- Eyeglasses (both reading and distance, if used)
- Chapstick
- Hair ties, bands, bobby pins
- Shaving essentials (personal razors, shaving cream)
- Personal-size mirror
- Pull-up briefs (if used)
- Male/female incontinence pads or panty lines (if used)
- Wet wipes
- Q-tips
- Container(s) to store toiletry items
- Hearing aids with extra batteries (if used)

What sort of clothing and shoes should I provide my loved one? How many pairs?

As described earlier, labeling everything is absolutely necessary to keep items where they belong. Make sure that belongings are clearly marked by yourself or the facility in a way that can withstand multiple washes. Either check those items periodically for fading labels or ask your loved one's CNA to check when they have a chance.

Bring at least a week's worth of loose-fitting, comfortable outfits to ensure your loved one has rotating items to wear while clothing is being laundered. Two pairs of comfortable shoes would also be ideal.

The most important items that families forget to bring are a pair of comfortable walking shoes and outer layers and jackets. Some facilities are air-conditioned, and if your loved one is someone who easily gets cold, they will appreciate a variety of sweaters or jackets to keep cozy in. Bras and belts are often forgotten, too!

Comfortable shoes (preferably a half size larger to make wearing easier) will go much further for your loved one than house slippers, flats, or dress shoes. If your loved one has trouble reaching down, slip-on or velcro strap shoes and a long-handled shoe horn will elevate their independence. It is important to remember that anyone with balance problems is at heightened risk of falling wearing anything other than supported, comfortable shoes.

Furthermore, if you can, laundering your loved one's clothes instead of having the facility do so can ensure that those items aren't misplaced. While laundry staff work tirelessly to return clothing where they belong, fading tags, untagged clothing, and illegible names are usually the culprit for clothing going missing.

What are some other items I could bring my loved one if they're staying long-term?

If your loved one's stay at a nursing facility is planned for the long-term, you may want to think beyond just essential comforts when it comes to making their stay more positive.

We all normally like a certain style of pillow: firm, soft, or somewhere in between. Bringing your loved one a pillow of their choosing would be so appreciated. In addition, a decorative or favorite blanket from home can spruce up a plain room and make them feel more at home.

A box of earplugs and an eye mask are some of the best items you can bring to encourage peaceful rest if deemed safe by your loved one's nurses. If your loved one can sleep with earplugs comfortably, this will be extremely beneficial to their sleep hygiene, as SNFs can be noisy at times. Furthermore, if your loved one has a roommate that likes to keep their light on into the wee hours of the morning, an eye mask will be extremely useful in blocking out unwanted light.

Watching TV and keeping up with the news is a major hobby for many older adults. If possible, bring your loved one wireless headphones that connect with their TV. This will allow them to listen to their favorite broadcasts and not compete with their neighbor's TV. For many, this makes a world of difference in their comfort and relaxation. You can collaborate with the maintenance supervisor to set this up.

If your loved one used any adaptive devices at home, such as a long-handled shoe horn, reacher, or mobility brace (i.e., knee brace), consider bringing these items in for them to encourage independence with getting dressed and moving around.

If your loved one has visual impairments, other adaptive devices from home that could be useful include magnifying glasses for reading, visual aids, and audiobook readers (with headphones).

PART THREE

Mental and Physical Well-Being

How do I ensure my loved one stays engaged in the nursing facility?

One of the biggest transitions I've seen individuals newly admitted into nursing facilities go through is the loss of routine and structure. Residents who were once sewers, dancers, hikers, and writers are in a new environment where carrying those hobbies out is much more challenging.

This doesn't mean all hope is lost, however. And if your loved one's stay in a nursing facility is planned for the long-term, this is an especially important area to prioritize in their care.

I have seen individuals prosper when they are provided with the things that give them meaning. Whether that means a headset with their favorite music, a collection of books in the genre of their preference, or crafts of their preferred variety, individuals who have something they love to do will often find solace in being able to continue these hobbies.

One resident, "Sue", loved knitting and was especially excited to prepare her Christmas gift one year: a knitted knapsack for every other resident in the facility. This was well-received because, without a purse, it can be hard to bring items along— especially if your hands are occupied by using a walker or wheelchair.

Sue's knapsacks were fashioned by many residents for a long time to come. She must have found great satisfaction in using her hobby for such a useful purpose.

Activities departments usually have a selection of crafts and hobbies that your loved one may be interested in. Check with the activities staff to see what items they have. If your loved one has a hobby that isn't accounted for, providing those items (i.e., knitting needles and yarn, Kindle or e-readers, laptops, specific books, or music) could mean the world to them. It is a gesture of, "*I care about your well-being, too, not only your essential needs.*"

You can also check with the activities department about any other services they provide, such as outings to local restaurants and malls. Some facilities even have pets that visit for those who love animals. Others have church services, musicians, and more.

Spontaneous visits are a good way to see if your loved one is keeping busy. Coming into your loved one deeply involved in a task versus sitting unoccupied could be a hint as to their level of engagement. If your loved one doesn't seem like they've found enough to do throughout the day, figure out why. It can be a very empowering conversation.

The most important thing is to ensure that your loved one has their hobbies around them. If they truly identify their only interest as watching television, make sure that their TV is working properly with access to the channels they enjoy. Ensure that a remote is provided. A pair of TV headphones would also be very useful!

What are some ways I can encourage the memory and orientation of my loved one?

If your loved one has a diagnosed cognitive impairment—such as dementia—or is just forgetful at times, it would help to provide a large print calendar to aid with day and time orientation. Calendars help an individual keep track of the passage of time, remember important dates, and recall appointments and visits.

A notepad could also help your loved one keep a log of interactions they've had, names of staff members they want to memorize, issues they're working on getting resolved, and even when they've taken medication. There are so many uses for blank notepads, and even better: a lot of pens and pencils to go with them!

Finding a clock that is large enough and easy to read will help your loved one remain aware of the time of day. Ensure the clock matches their needs (i.e., if your loved one is visually impaired, some clocks speak the time out when prompted). This is a simple fix and can aid in staying oriented and alert.

How can I personalize my loved one's space to make them feel more at ease?

In addition to belongings contributing to a sense of self, it is underestimated how important it can be to decorate your loved one's room with their favorite memories. This can be photos of family or even hobbies they enjoy (i.e., bowling or fishing). I've also seen many residents who like to keep cards from family and friends, reminding them that they are loved.

So often, I am moved by how much these physical artifacts matter to individuals in SNFs. They often use photos as a sense of pride (*"look at my grandson graduating!"*) and a way of being able to tell a story or experience that meant a lot to them (*"that is when I caught the biggest fish in my hometown!"*)

For those cognitively impaired individuals, labeling the back (or even front) of family photos with the names of loved ones can trigger memories and encourage positive reflection about their histories. Sometimes it's as simple as remembering a name that brings a pleasant memory back.

Decorating your loved one's space – however big or small it is – will make a lasting impression and remind them that they are loved and supported. Bringing a familiar blanket from home can make them feel at ease when going to bed at night. Think about those artifacts that we take for granted daily. They are the little influences that will encourage comfort and a sense of home—especially when accustoming to a new place.

What can I do if my loved one is dissatisfied with their roommate(s)?

Some of the best friendships I've seen forged in nursing facilities have been individuals who've shared a room, got to talking, and realized they have a lot in common. Beyond just getting along, if two people share the same set of desires (i.e., TV off by 9 pm), they are much more likely to be happy roommates.

One of the best things I've witnessed is when two individuals connect and get to talking late into the evening, recounting their life stories to each other, and sharing laughs. They can bond over their experiences. In an environment where things may initially feel so foreign, having the comfort of a friendly roommate can ease the inevitable transition.

Finding this type of connection can be hard, but it is not impossible. Everyone has different routines, and the staff tries to consider roommate compatibility when choosing a room for your loved one.

If you think back to a time you may have had a roommate, how you got along with that person probably made all the difference in your experience living there. That is why it is important to know that your loved one can request a room change if things aren't working out. The facility will try to accommodate the request as best as possible and consider the habits of new, potential roommates in an attempt to match the right individuals.

A room change means your loved one has to adjust to a new living area and new CNAs as well; however, if the roommate combination was not good, these adjustments can be well worth it.

If your loved one isn't able to voice their opinions for one reason or another, check with staff about your loved one's interactions — if any—with their roommate(s) and try to remain a passive and impartial observer when you are present to ensure that everyone seems comfortable and content.

Should I bring anything to encourage my loved one's mobility?

Usually, individuals living in nursing facilities have mobility challenges ranging from mild to severe. Residents often rely on mobility aids (i.e., walkers, canes, or wheelchairs) to get from point A to B. If your loved one is capable of standing and moving around safely, either by themselves or with someone, they have likely been assessed to determine which aid best serves their needs. They will usually be supplied with whatever aid is necessary.

If allowed by the facility, it is helpful that your loved one's mobility aid has a tag with their name and/or room number on it to ensure these items stay close by. This will also help it from becoming misplaced.

Wheelchairs and walkers benefit from having small baskets or bags to put belongings in when someone is on the go, but this isn't often provided by facilities I've worked in. This would be a wonderful addition to your loved one's mobility aid if you can supply it.

What can I do for my loved one if they are staying in bed too much?

If your loved one is mostly staying in bed, first check that there is not a medical reason that your loved one cannot get out of bed safely. If your loved one can tolerate sitting up, they can be transferred or mechanically lifted into a proper wheelchair to spend time up. There are mechanical lifts that allow an individual who cannot stand or transfer to be safely moved from one location to another.

Pressure sores are wounds that occur when there is prolonged and constant pressure over one area. They happen most often in individuals who are immobile or generally unable to reposition themselves (Bhattacharya & Mishra, 2015). Encouraging regular out of bed time for your loved one will decrease pressure in the areas that may constantly receive it from lying down. It will also allow your loved one the opportunity to observe new surroundings, get some fresh air, and encourage social interaction. [1]

A loved one with poor cognition or who is unable to speak may need you to advocate for getting out of bed, if necessary. Physical and occupational therapists are specialized in finding the safest way to help your loved one up. If possible, request PT or OT if you notice your loved one isn't as mobile as before or getting out of bed as frequently.

If your loved one is in a facility long-term, the rehabilitation team (PTs, OTs, and SLPs) may be familiar with them and can deduce what has changed in their abilities after conducting an evaluation. Check in with therapists or the director

---

[1] Being in a wheelchair for too long can have its risks for some individuals, too. If your loved one isn't able to independently reposition themselves, they may need to be repositioned during certain intervals or avoid prolonged sitting. If possible, see if they can be evaluated by an occupational therapist for pressure-relief options and education.

of rehabilitation (DOR) around your loved one's progress if they are on therapy services. Their goal is also to help maximize your loved one's independence and mobility.

If there are *medical limitations* affecting your loved one getting out of bed regularly, this will need to be closely monitored. If your loved one's vital signs are not stable, this will usually affect being able to sit up in a chair. For example, it is not advised to sit somebody up who is experiencing low blood pressure or who is experiencing a high resting heart rate. Should your loved one have issues in these areas, they may need to be monitored closely when/if they are stable enough to sit in a chair.

If there are *physical limitations* affecting your loved one getting out of bed regularly (i.e, sitting completely upright is too painful for their back), alternative seating options can be considered (i.e., reclining chairs that elevate the feet and recline the back). If capable of having therapy services, ask for an occupational therapy referral to conduct a seating assessment if your loved one is having issues sitting in a standard chair. There are many options!

Finally, if your loved one is in a fragile medical state and simply cannot safely leave their bed regularly, the team will need to evaluate the best way to prevent pressure sores in bed. An example is the use of an *alternating pressure air mattress*. This type of mattress takes pressure off individual areas of the body every few minutes to keep one area from sustaining pressure for too long.

If your loved one is mostly in bed, you can discuss any pressure-related concerns with their care team. Preventing pressure sores is a multidisciplinary effort and one of everyone's top priorities. Remember: prevention is best when it comes to skin issues. With that being said...

How can I prevent my loved one from acquiring a pressure sore?

Immobility is just one of the factors that contribute to pressure sores. Nurses typically conduct an assessment called the Braden Scale with any new resident, which takes into account risk factors that contribute to pressure sores. These factors include (but are not limited to): a person's ability to reposition themselves, how much moisture their skin is exposed to, their diet, and whether an individual is mostly in bed, in a chair, or can walk (Lyder, 2008).

Here are some strategies to help your loved one prevent pressure sores from happening in the first place:

- **If your loved one isn't able to reposition themselves**, they should be repositioned at regular intervals. Your loved one may also need to be considered for pressure-relief items when out of bed (i.e., special seating cushions).
- **If your loved one's nutritional needs aren't being met for one reason or another**, they should be evaluated by a registered dietician for recommendations.
- **If your loved one is incontinent**, they should be changed regularly and/or have a toileting schedule to prevent moisture on the skin for too long.
- **If your loved one requires a lot of help out of bed but can tolerate sitting**, they should be lifted into a wheelchair with appropriate cushioning.
- **If your loved one has new or recent trouble turning in bed or repositioning**, they should be seen by physical therapy (if possible) to address these concerns and figure out how to improve their skill or modify the surroundings.

Since prevention is key when it comes to pressure sores, ask your loved one's team about what is being done to prevent them. This will be an important area to keep track of, especially if your loved one is unwilling or unable to leave the bed regularly.

Why doesn't my loved one have bed rails?

Bed rails come in a lot of different sizes and help a person by giving them something to hold onto while trying to get out of bed or turning side to side. They can certainly be a useful aid in mobility and benefit plenty of residents. Some also feel that, because hospital-style beds tend to be narrow, they can prevent an individual from falling out of them unintentionally.

While it may not seem obvious, there are risks involved when deciding to place bed rail(s) for a resident to use. Potential risks of bed rail use include skin bruising, cuts, and scrapes, as well as injury if a body part gets caught between the bed and railing. Bed rails can also be viewed as a restraint, as they can sometimes block an individual who can leave their bed independently from being able to do so (Center for Devices and Radiological Health, 2010).

According to the FDA, residents with problems of incontinence, sleep, memory, pain, and uncontrollable body movements are the most important to consider when determining the use of bed rails (Center for Devices and Radiological Health, 2010). Different facilities have varying policies that dictate bed rail use. It is important that, if you have concerns, you discuss this with your loved one's nurse or therapist. You can also ask about other strategies that the staff are employing if you are afraid that your loved one may fall out of bed.

Some questions you can ask include:
- *Can my loved one be assessed for safe use of railings?*
- *How frequently is someone checking in on my loved one?*
- *Is my loved one's bed being kept lower to the ground?*
- *Is my loved one requesting to use the restroom? Is someone helping them? Is my loved one having any issues getting out of bed without a rail? Do they need a rail to turn side to side?*
- *Are there other options to help my loved one get out of bed more independently?*

Even more important than checking in with staff is checking in with your loved one. Determine if they are fearful of falling out of bed or are having trouble repositioning or getting up without a bed rail. If your loved one is on physical or occupational therapy, you can speak with their therapists to determine if there are other ways to prevent falls (things like positioning aids and having a toileting schedule can help).

What can be done to prevent my loved one from having falls?

One in four Americans over the age of 65 falls every year (National Council on Aging, 2021). As you may know, falls happen all the time with children, who are usually able to get up and brush themselves off. With older adults, however, these falls can result in life-changing injuries and traumas. This is why preventing falls from ever happening is absolutely imperative.

There are so many factors that can increase a person's risk for falling. Here are just a few:
- Lack of restful sleep
- Decreased vision
- Cognitive impairments

- Confusion or delirium
- Urge incontinence
- Dehydration
- Spills on floor/objects on the ground
- New medication
- Muscle weakness or decreased strength
- Sensory impairments (i.e., numbness on feet)
- Vertigo or dizziness
- Sudden drops in blood pressure or low blood pressure

Since reasons for falling are so wide-spread, *fall prevention* is a multidisciplinary effort that requires intervention from virtually everyone: nurses, CNAs, doctors, therapists, and more.

If your loved one is deemed at high risk for falling, it is important to understand why. Knowledge of the root cause(s) can make a large difference when it comes to preventing future falls.

You may also want to be aware of strategies employed to prevent falls. If your loved one is having falls while getting up or walking, they may require more frequent check-ins from staff to offer assistance. They would also benefit from an assessment by rehab professionals, if possible.

Falls related to bathroom visits

If your loved one is getting up to the bathroom without assistance but needs it, you may want to provide them reminders to wait for staff and/or call for help before it becomes urgent, since they'll need to account for the time it takes for staff to arrive. An occupational therapist (OT) may also be appropriate at this point to assess the safest way to help your loved one independently use the restroom.

Falls related to cognitive impairments

Loved ones with dementia or other cognitive impairments who are unable to safely walk on their own may attempt to get up by themselves. Often, they are not aware of their impairments and therefore fall trying to move around as they are used to doing. Increasing supervision and/or changing a loved one's room to one that is more highly visible by staff can ensure greater assistance is present for your loved one's safety. OTs can also assess your loved one's living space for modifications to prevent falls (i.e., placing non-skid treads on the ground or clearing the environment of fall hazards or obstructions).

Falls related to bed

If your loved one is falling out of bed, OTs and PTs can assess what sort of positioning devices or bolsters can assist with ensuring your loved one is resting more safely. They may educate nursing staff about how to best position your loved one in bed to prevent falls. Staff may also need to constantly ensure that the height of the bed is low to the ground. Some facilities may also introduce fall pads near the bedside to prevent injury if other methods have not been successful.

Falls related to sitting up in a chair

Those who primarily use wheelchairs can also be at risk for falling. This tends to happen if they're unable to reposition on their own and begin sliding down in the chair or by falling asleep and falling forward. An OT can help determine the safest chair for your loved one as well as how long they should remain in it at a time. They can then educate your loved one's nurses and CNAs on their findings.

Falls related to waiting for help

Unfortunately, sometimes a resident falls because they are restless or awaiting help. Long wait times are a battle that facilities must tackle to ensure that residents at risk for falling aren't resigning to getting up on their own. Decreasing the time spent waiting for assistance takes the combined effort of an entire facility and ensuring enough staff are present to handle the needs of residents.

What sort of mental health services are available for my loved one?

Most facilities refer to psychological services when signs of depression or other mental health concerns are noticed. Psychologists that visit facilities have a list of residents they are seeing and a description of what they were referred for. Psychologists can also request a visit by a psychiatrist (a medical doctor who can prescribe medications) if they feel that is needed.

In a facility, the people that usually know your loved ones the most are direct care staff, including CNAs, nurses, and rehabilitation professionals. These individuals spend most of their time with your loved one and are involved regularly in their care. They may be the first to notice when something seems off. If a change is subtle, however, it may only be you and/or other family members that detect a problem.

Psychologists working in nursing facilities can be some of the most helpful resources in your loved one's journey; however, visits can be shorter if they are managing a high caseload. This is by no fault of their own.

If your loved one has been followed by a psychologist or psychiatrist in the past, or if their psychological needs don't appear to be met, it would be best to ask for assistance with setting up an outpatient appointment, if possible. This would allow your loved one to see a mental health professional already familiar with their needs or who specializes in their area of concern.

Does my loved one have access to an optometrist and vision services?

Nursing facilities work with optometrists who visit at certain intervals and conduct eye exams. They can request for new prescriptions and address any vision-related concerns your loved one may have. You can request to have your loved one seen by the optometrist during their next facility visit. In my experience, it is the social services staff that handles these scheduled visits.

Does my loved one have access to dental care? How can they maintain their oral health?

Oral care is extremely important to health and well-being and something we want to ensure our loved ones are partaking in.

Each nursing facility works with a dentist, and dental consultations can be provided for them. You can request to speak with the dentist related to any concerns you have and how they believe your loved one's oral care routine should look.

The consequences of poor oral care can be detrimental: it has been linked to a greater risk of nursing-home acquired pneumonia (Quagliarello et al., 2005).

If your loved one is unable to follow a routine for themselves, you may want to ensure one is set up and that it is prioritized. [2]

My loved one sees a podiatrist. Will they have access to one in the facility?

Podiatrists make regular visits to facilities. A little known fact is that if your loved one is diabetic, they can only have their toenails clipped by a qualified nurse or podiatrist. This may cause some discomfort, as nobody likes growing their toenails out too long. In my experience, you can speak with the social services department to have your loved one added to the podiatry list so that they can be seen during the podiatrist's next visit. You can inquire about when that will be as well as any insurance coverage questions you may have.

Why is my loved one only given a certain texture of food? Why is their water thickened?

Your loved one is assigned a diet based on recommendations from medical professionals. Many conditions can affect a person's ability to safely swallow certain textures. If your loved one has swallowing difficulties or cognitive issues, a speech-language pathologist (SLP) will likely be involved in determining what textures are safest for them.

Dietary restrictions are in place for your loved one's safety. If your loved one is on a thickened liquid or softened texture for solid foods, this is likely due to a SLP's judgment of them needing this texture to prevent medical complications.

---

[2] Of note: If your loved one has dentures, they should be cleaned regularly and removed during sleep to prevent aspiration pneumonia, especially in the very elderly age group (85 and older) (Iinuma et al., 2014).

A SLP studies swallowing on an advanced level and does not want to keep individuals on alternate textures (such as pureed) unless they are needed for safety. They will often continue to conduct trials until they've settled upon the safest diet at that given time.

Understandably, many individuals that need to be placed on a soft or pureed diet are not happy about these restrictions. Fortunately, a lot of residents feel better if they are at least able to eat preferred foods in these textures.

I once had a resident's family puree all of their favorite foods and bring them their meals every single day. They also checked in with the SLP regarding what types of food are already considered puree (such as smooth mashed potatoes) and found the best pureed foods around. That resident was pretty happy and definitely well-fed!

Check with your loved one's SLP and dietary supervisor about what is safe to bring from home if they are on an altered diet. It could make a world of difference.

What is aspiration and aspiration pneumonia? Why should I know about it?

Aspiration occurs when foreign materials enter the lungs, including food, vomit, saliva, and liquids. These particles are normally swallowed into the stomach, but some conditions (such as Parkinson's disease, dementia, and stroke) can affect the way an individual swallows them.

Aspiration can lead to pneumonia, which is a swelling or infection of the lungs. Pneumonia can usually be treated with antibiotics; however, it is important to know if aspiration is the suspected cause. If it is, the doctor may order a swallow evaluation to determine the safest diet textures for your loved one. This is to avoid recurrent pneumonia episodes and the chance for greater health problems.

If your loved one has been diagnosed with aspiration pneumonia, they will have aspiration *precautions*. Other conditions can also lead to your loved one needing aspiration precautions in place. Aspiration precautions can include (but are not limited to): keeping your loved one's head of bed elevated 30 to 45 degrees at all times, maintaining upright sitting while eating and for some duration after, and following specific orders made by the speech-language pathologist (SLP). These orders can be a certain way of eating or drinking (i.e., not using straws for drinking or alternating a bite of food with a sip of liquid).

If your loved one is at risk for aspiration or has experienced aspiration-related pneumonia, speak with their SLP to ensure you are aware of what recommendations they have made to prevent future episodes.

How does my loved one leave the facility for appointments or other needs?

Although someone staying in a nursing facility can have most of their care handled from within, there may be a need to leave the SNF for some services, such as dialysis, MRIs, specialty visits, and more.

Work with the social services director(s) to devise a transportation plan for when your loved one needs to leave for appointments or visits. If your loved one is mobile and safe to transfer in and out of a car, you may be able to choose to provide transportation yourself.

Even if your loved one primarily uses a wheelchair, you can borrow a wheelchair from the facility so long as they can safely transfer in and out of a car into it. At your destination, you'll be able to assist by pushing their wheelchair for them, if necessary.

If you are unsure whether your loved one can safely transfer into your car, you can request that therapy first assesses their safety (if on therapy services).

Paratransit Services

If transferring into a car isn't an option, there is another way. The Americans with Disabilities Act (ADA) requires transit agencies to provide paratransit services to those individuals who are unable to access standard bus or rail transport due to physical, visual, cognitive, or other impairments. Most individuals staying in a nursing facility are qualified for this service. Qualification will usually require an interview process.

Once qualified, you or your loved one will have to call in advance to schedule a ride and return trip to and from a destination. The best part is that these services can accommodate those with wheelchairs and other mobility aids. Since these adaptive rides have a wheelchair lift, your loved one won't need to leave their seat at all!

Medical Transport

If your loved one is medically fragile, the only safe option may be private medical transportation. These services are for individuals who cannot safely sit upright in a wheelchair for long periods and therefore need to use a gurney or stretcher to get to an appointment, lying flat. They are also for individuals who may require close medical watch while being transported to their appointments.

These medical transportation services can incur some sort of fee, depending on your loved one's insurance.

If your loved one requires this type of transport, check with the social services department about the options they have as well as any costs associated.

Even though my loved one lives in the facility, can they leave for visits?

At facilities I have worked in, a resident can request to leave the facility "on pass". This means a loved one picks them up and takes them home, to a restaurant, or any place of their choosing. The pass is given by the facility physician and will include how many hours they are allowed to leave for (i.e., 4 or 8). The physician will evaluate a resident's health and medical needs when determining if and when they can leave on pass.

If going out on pass is an option for your loved one, consult with the rehabilitation department to determine your loved one's mobility needs and what you can do to ensure their safety while they are out and about.

Note: If you aren't able to safely help your loved one into a car, this doesn't mean you can't schedule outings! Paratransit services sometimes allow for a "buddy pass",meaning you can ride with them to a destination. If your loved one does not qualify for this, you can schedule a paratransit ride for your loved one somewhere and just meet them there for your outing!

Many families opt for this method to bring their loved ones home for the holidays. It is a joyous occasion for a resident who gets to go home and share the warmth of a holiday or event with their loved ones. Simply being able to sit at a dinner table with family is something they have shared excitedly with me time and time again. [3]

---

[3] Due to the current COVID-19 pandemic, passes of this nature are on suspension at the time of this guide. Unfortunately, it is uncertain when it may be possible again; however, it is good to know that, when it is safe to do so, you can ask about your loved one's options for visiting home!

PART FOUR

Rehabilitation and Discharge Planning

Short-term Stays

How does rehabilitation assist my loved one to return home?

Occupational therapists (OTs), physical therapists (PTs), and speech-language pathologists (SLPs) work to improve your loved one's functional abilities with the objective of helping them return home as safely as possible.

Therapists will begin by conducting evaluations of your loved one's abilities within a few days of their arrival in a SNF. Almost always, this will be both OT and PT. If your loved one has concerns in the areas of language, speech, cognition, or swallowing, an SLP will also be involved.

During their assessments, therapists will gather information from your loved one (or close family) regarding how they were functioning at home and what will be needed to safely return. For example, a PT seeing your loved one may ask if they needed help getting out of bed before and who assisted them. They may be curious if your loved one needed a cane or walker to get around the house. Meanwhile, an OT may ask if your loved one needed help with tasks such as bathing, toileting, and getting dressed.

An SLP may want to know if your loved one was able to communicate effectively before, faced memory challenges, or had any difficulty chewing and swallowing certain textures, depending on what they are assessing for.

Once a *prior level* is established, therapists develop goals for what they'd like your loved one to be able to achieve and work with them on those *goals* using different treatment approaches. During the treatment process, physical therapy assistants (PTAs), occupational therapy assistants (OTAs), and occasionally speech-language pathology assistants (SLPAs) may also work with your loved one and are wonderful at providing targeted interventions. The hope is that with their skills, your loved one will be able to achieve the goals necessary to return home safely.

What can I do to prepare for my loved one that is returning home?

Preparing for your loved one's safe return home becomes a priority the moment they enter a nursing facility. In medical jargon, this is referred to as *discharge planning*. Most disciplines (especially therapy and social services) want to know what is already available to a person at home so that they can establish realistic goals and work on providing equipment or the necessary help to ensure a smooth transition.

One thing to make sure to ask for your loved one is home health therapy (occupational, physical, and/or speech-language pathology) if they presently need those services in the facility. The rehabilitation process is a continuum of care and does not just stop when a person goes home. Often, a person will need to continue to see rehab professionals upon leaving to ensure a safe transition back into their familiar environment.

Occasionally, I've witnessed the importance of speech-language pathology in the continuum of rehab go unrecognized or forgotten. You may find that you need to advocate for including a speech-language pathologist on the list of services coming home with your loved one, if it's needed.

If possible, share photos or videos of your loved one's home set-up with their PTs and OTs at the nursing facility. Photos of stairs in the front of a home, bedrooms, and bathroom set-ups are very appreciated by rehab staff. This will allow them to simulate and practice skills that will be essential for them to safely navigate their unique environments.

PTs and OTs will recommend equipment (called *durable medical equipment* or DME) your loved one will need to safely return home. A lot of this equipment can be covered by insurance, but certain items may not be. Check with social services about what may not be covered, and ask your loved one's therapists for alternative ways of retrieving those items. In many places, there are local programs and nonprofits that provide medical equipment for free or heavily-discounted prices.

Therapists can conduct something called *caregiver training* with you or whoever may be involved in your loved one's care before they are discharged home. This can be done in-person or virtually, and involves the therapist educating you on the best ways to help your loved one once they're back home. It can involve suggestions (i.e., how to remind your loved one to use a walker safely) and training (i.e., how to transfer your loved one from a bed to a wheelchair or a commode). Caregiver training will also allow you to ask therapists any questions you have about helping your loved one at home.

In addition, the therapy team may also make recommendations for modifications (i.e., installing a grab bar in the tub, purchasing a ramp). Some therapy departments conduct home evaluations, where a therapist visits your loved one's home within a few days of their expected discharge. The individual is present with the therapist and goes about their routines: moving around in the bathroom, bedroom, and living spaces. This allows the therapist to see the individual in their normal environment before making final recommendations.

Try to avoid making any drastic changes until advised by the team. While the intent is good, sometimes what seems practical may not be exactly what your loved one specifically needs. Hold off until you've been given a clear picture of what changes need to be made!

What should I do if my loved one needs more assistance than I can provide?

When planning for your loved one to return home, you will be advised by the care team about how much assistance your loved one may require for certain tasks, as well as the amount of supervision they need for their own safety. This can range from a few hours a week to 24/7 care.

For those loved ones requiring more care, I have seen family members split caregiving duties. For example, if a resident normally lives with her daughter, but her daughter works daytime hours, another family member would be present during the day until evening. Hired caregivers are also a common option for providing care when no one else is available.

If your family is unable to manage the amount of care your loved one needs, the social services director will work with you on providing options for privately hiring a caregiver, as well as applying for state-sponsored at-home caregiving services (if your loved one qualifies). These programs provide a specific amount of caregiving services monthly free of charge. These hours are decided after the program reviews your loved one's needs.

If qualified for these government-sponsored programs, a list should be provided to you or your loved one of potential caregivers, who can then be interviewed for compatibility. You can also elect a family member or friend to be compensated for being your loved one's designated caregiver under this program.

Some home health agencies also provide a home health aide to visit for a while after your loved one returns home. The aide can assist with areas your loved one may still help with, such as bathing. In my experience, this service is usually a few days a week, for several hours a day. It is important to know that home health aides are not long-term, consistent caregivers and are meant only to assist with the transition process. You may have to look into hiring a caregiver if help is needed beyond the time they are provided.

Do not be alarmed if you don't feel you do not have all the pieces together. Discharge planning can take time to truly create a working plan for your loved one.

What options are available if my loved one isn't able to safely return home?

If your loved one's plan is to return home and you've exhausted all options or possibilities, there are lower levels of care that your loved one can consider, such as board and care homes and assisted living facilities.

Board and care facilities are licensed and regulated homes that provide 24-hour staff and assistance with daily tasks, such as bathing, medication management, and meal prepping. Every board and care facility is different and can offer varying levels of help. Board and care facilities are usually personal homes meant for adults who need assistance that are medically stable enough not to require a nursing facility.

Assisted living facilities (or ALFs) are meant for older adults who require custodial care (i.e., dressing, bathroom use, or bathing care) but do not require around-the-clock nursing care found in SNFs. ALFs are usually residential style, with each individual having their own rooms. ALFs will provide meal, laundry services, and medication management; however, different ALF stays may cost differently depending on the level of services needed. For example, some of the residents I worked with cited paying more for an ALF stay if they needed services like transfer assistance or bathing.

Discuss these options with your loved one. If your loved one decides an alternate living arrangement needs to be made, remember that this can be a very emotional and difficult thing for them to process. Many individuals fear the idea of being unable to return home— and rightfully so. The hope is that an alternative living arrangement can be found that satisfies both your loved one's desire for comfort and a sense of home. Assist them through the process however you can and seek guidance for them if needed. Oftentimes, the social services director can be a great resource with this process.

Long-term Stays

Why isn't my loved one on rehab anymore? When will they see a therapist again?

One concern you may have if your loved one is transitioning to long-term care is the fear that they will no longer receive exercise or mobility once therapy has stepped out of the picture.

Something to be aware of is that therapy does not remain involved with a resident indefinitely, unlike nursing care. Usually, when a rehab professional is working with someone, they are progressing them toward greater independence, ensuring they are not going to experience decline, and/or finding ways to maintain their current level of function.

While therapy can be very useful in maintaining function (i.e., performing exercises to not lose arm strength), it is often not a reason to continue seeing an individual forever. [1]

If your loved one's stay is long-term, they will typically be seen by therapy services again if there is a noted decline in their functioning. For example, newfound trouble in your loved one's ability to walk or transfer into a wheelchair may require a physical therapy assessment, while a decline in your loved one's ability to dress themselves or use the bathroom may indicate the need for occupational therapy.

Furthermore, if your loved one begins to experience a cognitive decline or starts to experience trouble swallowing or managing certain foods/liquids, a speech-language pathology evaluation may be in order.

One thing to note is that if your loved one is having a new problem, it's important to rule out any possible medical causes. Certain infections and illnesses will manifest in the older adult population with symptoms like increased confusion, delirium, difficulty swallowing, decreased mobility, and more. Ensure that your loved one is also assessed by the medical team if experiencing a functional decline.

If your loved one has Medicare Part B, therapy services are covered under this insurance for long-term residents needing therapy. Once a resident is on therapy services, their deficits will be identified, and treatments will be designed

---

[1] In 2013, a settlement occurred as a result of *Jimmo v. Sebelius*. In this lawsuit, it was determined that, under Medicare coverage, an individual's therapy services are not dependent on whether they make progress, but rather, whether services are needed to not experience a set-back. That is, if one can prove that an individual requires skilled services to prevent decline, this is sufficient to provide care. It must be clear why an individual needs therapy services, and why these services cannot be provided by other staff (i.e., nursing).

to either re-establish independence or find other ways to perform tasks. Your loved one will remain in rehab services as long as the professional treating them believes they continue to make progress or benefit from it.

But PT, OT, and SLP are not the only sources of exercise, function, and mobility available in your loved one's journey. It is important to understand not only the role of these rehab services, but also of restorative nursing (RNA) programs and functional maintenance programs (FMP) as well. These services can keep your loved one engaged and functional when they are not actively being seen by therapy.

Most facilities have RNA programs designed to maintain a resident's function for longevity, so this is an important area to consider when selecting a facility for long-term care. You may want to ask your loved one's facility about how their specific restorative programs are run.

It may help to paint a picture of the cycle of therapy by providing an example. Here, "Mary" begins having trouble at mealtime. Her CNA notices and informs the charge nurse. The charge nurse then communicates this with the rest of the team, who refer Mary to OT:

An occupational therapist (OT) evaluates Mary and finds that she is experiencing issues with her fine motor coordination, or the control in her hands to hold smaller objects. The OT begins a therapy program to assist Mary with her coordination and introduces adaptive equipment, such as spoons and forks with built-up handles, for easier gripping. In this example, the OT is working on both restoring function (better fine motor coordination) as well as providing adaptations to ensure Mary will not experience any more decline (using built-up utensils).

You might wonder what will happen to Mary once she is off therapy. This is when the restorative nursing program or functional maintenance program comes into play.

How do I ensure my loved one maintains their abilities when they are not on therapy?

What happens after therapy is no longer in the picture is a big area of concern for many loved ones, and rightfully so. Nobody wants to see their loved one decline in their abilities. Per federal guidelines, a facility must ensure that each resident receives the necessary care and services *"to attain or maintain the resident's highest practicable physical, mental, and psychosocial well-being"* (U.S. Centers for Medicare & Medicaid Services, n.d.).

Restorative nursing programs are created by rehab professionals (OTs, PTs, or SLPs) and carried out by trained nursing staff (restorative nursing assistants, also called RAs or RNAs). RNAs are often CNAs (certified nursing assistants) trained to implement these programs. Therapists create RNA *goals* for either maintenance or progress of a certain skill. The intervention approach can be guiding your loved one through an exercise or even providing appropriate cueing to perform a task independently (i.e., self-feeding or dressing). The *frequency* (how many days a week) of this program is determined by the therapist creating it. RNA staff are also trained to monitor for progress or decline in the area they are working on.

Going back to "Mary" as an example again:

Once Mary's OT has determined she can successfully feed herself again, she begins to design a restorative program for the RNAs to carry out. The OT's RNA program includes that the RNA should continue to perform fine motor activities five days a week, as well as check in with Mary during lunchtime to ensure she is still doing okay using the adaptive equipment. Mary trains the RNA on the techniques that help Mary, as well as the equipment to make sure it is being provided to her at mealtime. The OT also shows the RNA how to best position Mary during mealtimes. The OT then discharges Mary from therapy, and the RNA begins to carry out the plan.

Restorative programs can be made for all sorts of areas; they can involve strengthening and range of motion exercises, assisting with transfers, walking, applying and removing splints on a schedule to prevent contractures, assisting with grooming and dressing activities, providing swallowing techniques at mealtime, maintaining bowel and bladder routines and much, much more.

Should Mary's RNA notice a change in her ability to feed herself, she will bring that to the therapist's attention to once again assess her for needs. Therefore, the relationship between rehab and the RNA is a close one: they are often communicating about residents who are on RNA programs for new needs they may have.

Similarly, a functional maintenance program (FMP) is one that is designed to prevent a decline in an individual. These typically involve less skilled care. An FMP can be carried out by a CNA who is already present to provide care, such as stretching or basic self-care. An FMP could include having a resident dress themselves or providing range of motion to the arms and legs on a regular basis during normal care. The goal here is to prevent declines in function. Similar to RNA, a resident on an FMP can be reassessed by a therapist should the nursing staff notice a decline occurring.

It is vital to understand the roles of therapy, restorative nursing programs, and functional maintenance programs in your loved one's care, as these are measures to ensure that they are able to continue functioning at the highest of their abilities. Check in with your loved one's facility's rehab director (DOR) or nursing director (DON) regarding their specific programs or if you have any concerns about your loved one's functional abilities.

PART FIVE

Advocacy and the Complaint Process

What rights does my loved one have while staying in a nursing facility?

The Nursing Home Reform Law passed in 1987 intends to improve the quality of care for nursing home residents across the United States. Under it, nursing facilities must work to protect the rights of their residents, as well as provide dignity and personal choice. Any facility that chooses to participate in Medicare or Medicaid must adhere to these rights.

Some examples of residents' rights include:

- Right to privacy
- Right to be fully informed
- Right to be free from neglect and punishment
- Right to reasonable accommodations
- Right to participate in one's own care
- Right to make a complaint

Each facility provides a new resident with a copy of these rights. These are important to hold onto if ever they need to be referenced (U.S. Centers for Medicare & Medicaid Services, n.d.).

Care Plans

Another thing to take note of is that a nursing facility must develop a plan of care (or care plan) for your loved one's stay. These are essentially written guidelines for how the facility will take care of your loved one's individual needs. Care plans involve instructions for targeting a specific concern (i.e., weight loss or skin issues). The aim is to have an organized way of managing and documenting all interventions being made to address your loved one's needs.

For example, a plan of care to reduce falls in a less-mobile resident that is getting out of bed unsupervised could be:

- Frequent staff check-ins
- Assisting the resident to the restroom frequently
- Providing leisure activities to promote engagement and decrease boredom

It is important to know that your loved one also has the right to involve family or friends in their plan of care and can seek family council regarding their needs while they stay within a nursing facility (U.S. Centers for Medicare & Medicaid Services, n.d.).

This is by no means a comprehensive overview as to what rights your loved one has within a nursing facility. Please consult with a legal expert or local nursing home advocacy group if you have more specific questions regarding your loved one's rights within a facility.

How are nursing homes monitored for the care they provide?

F-tags are federal regulations that govern long-term care facilities in the United States. Each F-tag bears a number that corresponds with a specific regulation. For example, F-757 refers to a facility having a *"Drug Regimen [that] is Free From Unnecessary Drugs"*. This means that the medications your loved one is receiving should only include those drugs that are necessary for them to take (U.S. Centers for Medicare & Medicaid Services, 2020).

F-tags are used by every state's Department of Health and the Centers for Medicare and Medicaid Services (CMS) to evaluate the care delivered to residents in nursing facilities. [1]

All nursing facilities must undergo annual surveys by their state's Department of Health. These surveyors are looking into many areas of care to determine whether that facility is up to standards, including thorough record keeping, good quality of care being given, and maintenance of proper infection control. Nursing homes that receive a violation of an F-tag are in breach of that specific code. Those facilities can then be subject to penalties and fines ranging in severity.

In addition, the Department of Health can also make impromptu visits into a nursing facility when a complaint has been made and an investigation is needed. This will involve interviewing, chart reviewing, observation, and more. Regulatory action can be taken if needed.

How can I check in on my loved one's care?

The best way to ensure your loved one is receiving quality care is by being an active visitor or by having someone visit regularly. Not surprisingly, residents with advanced dementia who are not visited have been found to have worse quality of care (Grabowski & Mitchell, 2009).

The best sign you can get about your loved one's care is how their needs are met when you are not around to advocate for them. That is why I recommend

---

[1] For your purposes, it may not be necessary to know what the individual F-tags are; however, it can be reassuring to just be aware that there is a system of how the federal and state governments monitor care within nursing facilities.

visiting unannounced to check in on how your loved one's treatment is going when you are not expected.

I also encourage a periodic visit during every shift that visitors are allowed to observe how treatment is occurring at all hours. As staff usually rotate every shift, the culture can be completely different at different times of the day or night.

How often should I visit my loved one?

Among all the residents I have worked with, I've found that those with regular visits and phone calls from loved ones seem to have the most comfortable transitions into a nursing facility. There appears to be a difference in the quality of life of residents who are regularly contacted by those who care about them.

While I've seen those with frequent family visits prosper, every family is different. Of course, you need to factor in your personal life and visit at a rate that works for you. The rule of thumb is clear, however: visit as often as you comfortably or reasonably can.

There is a certain excitement that comes over a resident who is expecting a visit from their loved one. One resident in particular was always overjoyed and up early to prepare. She was beaming from the visit long after her family had left and settled into their own homes.

Residents, without a doubt, tell me excitedly about family visiting during our therapy sessions (*"My son Jeremy came by and brought me flowers!"*). It seems to bring them the most joy out of anything, as well as a sense of comfort and pride.

In my experience, being checked-in regularly or visited by loved ones seems to have one of the largest impacts on the emotional well-being and adjustment of residents in a SNF. They find meaning in these visits more than we could ever imagine. They allow us to catch little changes before they become problematic. They provide a sense of consistency and something to look forward to.

Even if your loved one is cognitively impaired and may not remember your visit, your check-ins can have an impact more than you may be aware of. A resident going through short-term memory loss may often ask for their family member and is relieved – at least momentarily —when they can see a familiar face or hear a voice they can recall.

If your loved one is unable to speak on their own behalf, your visits allow you to be their voice to make sure their needs are being met and that they are as comfortable as possible. In fact, in some ways, your visits may be more important in this case.

If you are separated by a distance from your loved one's facility or cannot visit for one reason or another, try to appoint someone (another family member or a close friend) to be their visitor at whatever frequency you can achieve. Make regular phone calls if visits just aren't possible.

Remember: something is better than nothing! An effort to stay in contact is better than no effort at all. Keeping in touch can be one of the most meaningful ways to show your loved one that you care.

A Note on Visitation During the COVID-19 Pandemic

There is no doubt that COVID-19 has affected those in nursing homes, both physically from the infection and emotionally from isolation. At the time of writing this, visits are still restricted in most nursing facilities, with many facilities requiring appointments and social distancing protocols to ensure safety.

In the meantime, most family members are doing what they can to still show up in person. In most cases, this means visiting behind glass doors and windows.

From what I've experienced, residents in nursing facilities are experiencing loneliness and feeling cut off from the world due to the lack of outside contact. Try to visit in whatever way possible to show your loved one support, especially in this isolating time.

While visiting your loved one may be complicated at this time, tips within this guide should hopefully give you ways of supporting them—even from an unfortunate distance.

What if visiting isn't an option? How else can I check in?

In addition to communicating regularly with your loved one, checking in can be done in other ways. If you are not around often or your loved one cannot speak for themselves, remember: it is perfectly fine to make calls into the facility to ask how your loved one is doing and to get updates from staff.

A simple five-minute conversation can provide you with more information than you might think. Some example questions to ask staff when calling could be:

- *Did my loved one eat their meals today?*
- *Did my loved one complain of pain today?*
- *Did my loved one take all their medication?*
- *Did my loved one participate in therapy? (If applicable)*

- *Is my loved one awake and engaged? Do they seem tired?*
- *Did my loved one get out of bed today?*
- *Are there any items my loved one is running low on?*
- *Has my loved one requested for anything recently? Is there anything they need?*

Remember: for privacy reasons, certain personal and medical information can only be provided to those on your loved one's designated contact list.

While we continue to deal with the COVID-19 pandemic, socially distant visits have become common as a means of being able to physically see a loved one as well. Combined with phone check-ins, these visits can still have a positive and lasting impact on your loved one. It allows you to get a glimpse at how they are doing face-to-face, which is invaluable.

Recently, I saw a family setting up lawn chairs outside their mother's room. They called their mother by phone, who was inside the facility and able to have a conversation with them. She was able to witness her daughter and son-in-law smiling through the window, all while enjoying the beautiful orchids they had brought her.

The look on her face was indescribable: you could tell she felt loved. In addition to making their mother happy, this resident's family was also able to check in with her caregivers, nurse, and therapists around their mother's progress.

FaceTime and Skype

If you can acquaint your loved one with a tablet, phone, or laptop that allows for video calling, it is a great option for virtual check-ins. Video calls allow you to see each other's facial expressions when speaking and adds another layer of connection. This is a great way to gauge how your loved one is doing in a more thorough way than a voice call.

What are some signs to look for to ensure my loved one is receiving proper care?

Through my experiences, I have come upon a few indicators that someone may not be attended to as much as they should be. Remember that these are only signs, not proof that improper care is happening. They are areas to take mental notes on and to respond accordingly. Observing some of these signs can alert you to the potential for neglect, which will be discussed in an upcoming section.

Here are just a few cues that your loved one may not be attended to properly:

Your loved one has signs of poor hygiene [2]

Hygiene can be a major red flag as to the level of care being provided, as well as an indicator of elder neglect. Some signs that a resident may not have had thorough hygiene practices are:

- Unkempt or unwashed hair
- Nails that have not been cleaned or trimmed for long periods
- Clothing stains that do not appear fresh (or didn't appear after a meal)
- Teeth or dentures that appear to have visible food particles (again, not after mealtime)
- Stained or unclean bed sheets, particularly older appearing stains

---

[2] Poor hygiene can be a warning sign of neglect. Elder abuse (including neglect) will be addressed in a separate section and should be reviewed.

Your loved one's room is extremely messy (but not because of their own habits)

Nobody's room is perfectly tidy, but a particularly messy room can be a sign that it is not attended to regularly. Proper attention to a resident includes handling their belongings with care. If your loved one has organizers in place for different items and those items are nowhere to be found, there might be a problem with someone misplacing belongings or rushing through your loved one's care.

You cannot easily locate self-care items, such as toothbrushes and soap

Since hygiene is an extremely important part of every resident's daily routine, these items should be relatively easy to locate. Not finding a toothbrush or other basic essential care items in your loved one's room can be an indicator that these practices are not occurring as regularly as they should be. Check drawers for these items as well, as they may not be sitting in plain sight.

Staff do not seem to regularly check in with your loved one

Depending on the length of your visits, you should encounter at least one person checking in on your loved one. This can be something as simple as your loved one's CNA coming in to bring them a snack or an activity staff member handing out crossword puzzles.

Having regular check-ins by staff to ensure everything is okay is essential to the well-being of a person staying in a SNF. If you are visiting for longer than an hour or two without a single person coming into your loved one's room, this might be something to check in about.

Their call-light rarely seems to be answered in a reasonable amount of time

Using a call light is how a resident notifies their CNA or nurse that they need assistance with something. There is no perfect system where a call light is answered right away, no matter where you go. But your loved one should also feel that their call light is answered within a reasonable amount of time to address their needs (medication, bathroom use, etc). Have a discussion with the facility staff if your loved one's consistently experiencing long wait times to receive assistance.

Staff constantly seem extremely overworked or stressed

A nursing facility can be a fast-paced environment. Staff will be seen entering and exiting rooms often. In fact, there is probably something off if a facility doesn't seem busy at all.

On the other hand, if you constantly seem to notice overburdened and exhausted nursing staff, there is a chance that your loved one is being impacted by this. An overworked CNA may be juggling many patients she needs to provide care for. This minimizes the time she can spend with your loved one and, therefore, may unintentionally impact the level of care being given to them.

Your loved one has complaints, either directly or indirectly

While this seems obvious, it's important to observe how your loved one relates to their environment. Some people are less likely to complain but may make comments such as, "I wish I could brush my teeth daily" or "I can't remember the last time I had a shower."

Sadly, individuals undergoing some form of neglect may begin to feel that these basic activities are a luxury. Normalizing these conditions could result in your loved one complaining less to you or not at all. That is why it is important to pay attention to comments that can inform you of their normal care routines.

If you begin to tune into what your loved one is telling you, you can deduce an awful lot. But if your loved one is nonverbal, has dementia, or is otherwise unable to talk about their needs, you may need to rely solely on observation-based approaches to check in on your loved one's care.

What happens if my loved one's needs aren't being met or I need to make a complaint?

One of the key areas to empowering both you and your loved one is understanding what can be done should something go wrong. With complaints, there are several avenues you can choose to take, both internally within a facility and externally, with governing bodies and agencies. These agencies are set up to protect the rights of residents in long-term facilities. Let's begin by discussing the complaint process with the staff at your loved one's SNF.

Who do I complain to *within* a facility if something goes wrong?

As you've read through this guide, you hopefully now have an idea of the different departments in a SNF. If necessary, you can contact a specific department head to address concerns in that area (i.e., the director of rehab for therapy-related concerns or the dietary supervisor for meal-related concerns). As these individuals are trained in their specialties, they will likely have relevant solutions for your particular concerns.

If you would like to make a more formal complaint, every facility has a process of how these are handled. Check with your loved one's facility regarding their procedure and who complaints are addressed to. In my experience, it is typically the social services department that manages the complaint process.

Residents and their families also have the option to file a written grievance. This is a way to handle concerns in a more formal way, as the concerns are documented. The grievance process triggers the facility to investigate the complaint and attempt to find a resolution. These grievances are also discussed with the administrator, as well as the rest of the interdisciplinary team, if necessary.

If a problem can be addressed and solved within a facility, this is the best way to have changes made immediately. Throughout the years of working in SNFs, I have seen issues brought to the team taken seriously and, more time than not, action is taken to rectify the problem; however, it is also important to know where you can turn if a facility isn't handling your concerns appropriately.

Who do I complain to outside of a facility about my loved one's care? What is a Long-Term Care Ombudsman?

It is very important for anyone that has a loved one in a nursing facility to understand the role of a Long-term Care Ombudsman. This is an individual that is appointed to advocate for residents within a nursing facility. They can handle a resident's or family's concerns and investigate complaints made related to the violation of rights, suspected abuse, poor quality of care, and many other problems.

Start by locating the local ombudsman office in your area and have their information handy in case you ever need these services. If you have trouble locating this yourself, facilities are required to post the local office's number in a visible place. You can also ask about it directly.

Each state varies, but in California, there is also a dedicated Ombudsman CRISISline that is available to take calls 24-hours a day, 7-days a week. Check your state's specific Long-Term Care Ombudsman's office for information on what additional resources are available to your loved one.

Is there another avenue to file serious complaints?

If you are unable to have your needs met at the Ombudsman level, you are also able to contact your state's Department of Health office. Complaints made to the Department of Health are taken seriously and result in your state sending representatives to visit the facility. These individuals will gather artifacts and investigate the complaints made to the fullest extent possible. The investigation process can include interviewing staff and residents, reviewing charts, and observation. Depending on the case, investigations may take some time to reach a conclusion.

What if I feel nothing has been done to address my concerns by any of these resources?

It can happen. Unfortunately, some individuals find themselves unable to be helped by their loved one's nursing facility and by outside resources. With all options being exhausted, some individuals choose to take legal action against the facilities in which they have found their loved ones wronged. Litigation can take time and incur cost, but for some, it is a way to ensure no stones have been left unturned in a case of unsatisfactory, dangerous, or unacceptable issues that their loved one faced.

What are the different types of elder abuse?

Approximately 1 in 10 Americans over the age of 60 have experienced some form of elder abuse (National Council on Aging, 2021). Abuse is an extremely serious matter that should be treated as such. If you have any suspicions that your loved one is undergoing any of the following types of abuse, please take action:

Physical Abuse

Physical abuse may be the most commonly thought of when discussing abuse. It involves the intentional act of causing harm to another individual and can result in injury or trauma. Perhaps the most obvious sign of physical abuse is unexplained bruising.

Emotional/Psychological Abuse

This form of abuse can be more difficult to detect, as there aren't physical artifacts left behind like in physical abuse. Emotional or psychological abuse can entail verbal aggression, intimidation, and threats made to an individual.

Financial Abuse

Financial abuse involves the misuse of an elderly person's finances by another person. It can result in someone making transactions via the elderly person's account without their knowledge, stealing money, or engaging in financial fraud targeting senior citizens.

Neglect

Neglect is the failure to provide an individual with adequate care and safety needs. Passive neglect is important to understand, particularly with the elderly. It is when a caregiver fails to provide an older adult with basic necessities, such as food, clothing, shelter, and medical care.

Self-neglect

Some are confused by the idea of self-neglect. This is when an individual is unwilling or unable to handle their care or needs, such as bathing or regular meals, and are a danger to themselves because of this. It is seen less often within a SNF, as staff are usually monitoring a person's care and can provide help, but it is good to understand that it can happen among the elderly in the home environment.

Abandonment

Abandonment occurs in the elderly when an individual is left without the ability to obtain necessities, such as food, shelter, clothing, medical services, or safety. An example of this can include deserting an elderly family member at home who cannot otherwise care for themselves.

Sexual Abuse

Sexual abuse is fondling, touching, intercourse, or any sexual activity with an elderly individual who is either unable to consent (lacks capacity), or is unwilling, forced, or threatened into the act.

What are some warning signs of elder abuse?

It is important to be aware that improper care can be classified as neglect. Many times, abuse and neglect isn't reported directly to a loved one. Therefore, it is important to look at nonverbal cues that may be occurring. The following warning signs are taken from California's Adult Protective Services (APS) webpage:

- "Explanation for an injury is inconsistent with its possible cause
- Recent changes in the elder or dependent adult's thinking; seems confused or disoriented
- The caregiver is angry, indifferent, or aggressive toward the elder or dependent adult
- Personal belongings, papers, or credit cards are missing
- The elder appears hesitant to talk openly
- Lack of necessities, such as food, water, utilities, medications, and medical care
- The caregiver has a history of substance abuse, mental illness, criminal behavior, or family violence
- Another person's name added to the client's bank account or important documents, or frequent checks made out to cash" (Adult Protective Services, 2020)

In addition to these signs of abuse provided by APS, it is important to also consider signs of neglect within nursing homes. Neglect can be difficult to pinpoint because its results may, unfortunately, be manifested in many ways.

A few signs of neglect within a nursing home can include:

- Bed sores
- Unexplained weight loss (a sign of malnutrition)
- Dehydration
- Poor personal hygiene
- Newfound incontinence

Remember that abuse can occur in many ways. Remain vigilant if you have any suspicions, especially for a loved one who cannot speak for themselves.

Who do I contact if I suspect my loved one's been abused?

One study estimates that only 1 out of every 14 abuse cases is reported to the authorities. It is important to report abuse if you even *suspect* it has happened. [3]Adult Protective Services (APS) is the reporting body to contact to report a potential case of abuse. APS is available 24-hours a day, 7-days a week to receive calls and takes each case very seriously (National Council on Aging, 2021).

Every state has its own APS, and the service is handled by different departments. In California, APS is run by the Department of Social Services. In Texas, however, it is the Department of Family and Protective Services that APS works under.

---

3 A common misconception is that you need solid, concrete evidence that abuse occurred in order to contact APS. If there is a suspicion of suspected abuse, it is still best to report. At the end of the day, it is the job of APS to investigate a claim and determine whether, with as much evidence as is available, the abuse occurred or not. Your only responsibility lies in the reporting process.

One thing is common: every state has its own dedicated hotline. Refer to the Resources section of this guide for a list of every state's phone number for abuse reporting.

And of course, if any immediate danger is present, call 911 immediately.

What can I do if there is a change in my loved one's condition, health, or well-being?

If you notice a decline in either your loved one's mental or physical state, you should request to have them assessed by their nurse. Inform them of whatever you are noticing (*"Mom has a new cough and I am concerned that she's also very congested."*)

If, after this, you do not feel the concern has been appropriately addressed, you can also reach out to the nurse supervisor or even the director of nursing (DON).

Normally, the nurse will relay the *change of condition* to your loved one's facility doctor, nurse practitioner, or physician assistant. They can then address this change (i.e., ordering a lab test or prescribing a medicine), and nursing staff will continue to monitor your loved one for ongoing changes or improvement.

If you voice a concern about your loved one's health, feel confident making check-ins for progress. [4] Knowing updates can put you and your loved one at

---

[4] If you suspect a medical emergency (i.e., you've called or stepped in to visit and an emergency is happening), alert your loved one's nurse immediately or, if unable to find the proper contact, you can choose to call 911 on your own and direct them to the facility. Hopefully this is never the case with your loved one, but it is important to be aware that you have the right to call 911 for your loved one if you believe a medical emergency is happening.

ease that their concern is being addressed (i.e., asking your loved one's nurse: "Mom started taking cough medicine yesterday. Have you noticed an improvement?")

Request for a Specialist

If a lasting medical issue doesn't appear to resolve or becomes chronic, you may request that your loved one see a specialist. Some vital medical specialties you might want to be aware of, regardless of whether your loved one is in a facility or at home, include:

Neurology
This specialist treats dysfunction of the nerves and nervous system and works with individuals who experience seizures, nerve pain, chronic neurological diseases (such as multiple sclerosis), unexplainable neurological symptoms (such as tremors), disorders of sleep, and much more. In addition, if your loved one has a chronic or progressive neurological disease, it is important that they are followed by this specialist.

Physical Medicine and Rehabilitation
A PM&R doctor (or physiatrist) specializes in treating and rehabilitating conditions that affect an individual's performance and function. Rather than focusing solely on the "cure", these specialists are concerned greatly with improving quality of life and performance through means that are not only medication.

Pain Management
Pain specialists have advanced training in the management of both new and chronic pain conditions. When more common pain interventions are not enough to help an individual, a pain management doctor steps in to assess all

factors that could contribute to someone's pain. From this, they use a versatile approach to improve a person's quality of life and reduce suffering.

Gastroenterology

This specialist, often referred to as a GI doctor, deals with disorders of the stomach and intestines. As you may know, the digestive system is extremely important to our overall health and comfort, and chronic issues in this area will benefit greatly from seeing a specialist.

Geriatric Medicine

These specialists focus on the prevention and treatment of illnesses in the elderly. They have advanced knowledge of the aging process and often care for individuals living in nursing homes and/or hospitals.

Palliative Medicine

Palliative care specialists are composed of a team of doctors, nurses, and other professionals, all with the same focus: relieve suffering and improve quality of life. They are vital to those living with serious or chronic illness that makes day-to-day living difficult. For example, someone undergoing chemotherapy may want to seek a palliative specialist to address concerns of nausea, vomiting, fatigue, and other side effects of treatment.

Please note this list is not even close to comprehensive. In fact, there are over 135 specialties and subspecialties of medicine (Association of American Medical Colleges, 2021)!

Specialty appointments take place outside of the facility, which will require figuring out transportation. If you are uncertain how your loved one can get to their appointment, the social services department is the best place to start.

What is a "NOMNC"? What if I don't agree with my loved one's insurance terminating coverage for staying at a SNF?

NOMNC stands for Notice of Medicare Non-Coverage. If your loved one's stay is being paid for by Medicare, this is a notice provided if Medicare is choosing to terminate your loved one's coverage for staying at the facility. The reason for terminating coverage can vary, but it can mean that Medicare believes your loved one's care can be delivered at a lower level (i.e., at home with home health services).

Receiving a NOMNC notice can be stressful if there isn't already a plan in place for what your loved one will do after their facility stay. It is important to remember that receiving a NOMNC is an opportunity for you or your loved one to appeal for why they continue to require skilled coverage.

A successful appeal is made if you can prove that your loved one still requires the level of nursing and therapy care that is provided at a SNF. A few examples of NOMNC appeals could be:

- Your loved one still needs intensive therapy services to increase their physical independence needed to go home safely
- Your loved one continues to require around-the-clock supervision or care by licensed nurses because they are not medically stable enough for less help
- Your loved one does not yet have a safe plan for where they are going when leaving the nursing facility

A successful appeal will not result in a permanent extension, but it can delay the process and give you and your loved one time to determine the next step.

Remember that the discharge process for your loved one is not something that you must figure out alone as a family. There is always support available. Social services directors and case managers are specialized in handling concerns and discussing various options around discharge planning. Meanwhile, the rehab department can provide invaluable advice on what assistance and equipment are needed for the next steps.

A NOTE ON COVID-19

At the time of writing this guide, the world is experiencing an unprecedented pandemic in the form of Coronavirus Disease 2019 (COVID-19). It is known that COVID-19 affects the elderly disproportionately when compared to younger individuals (Williamson et al., 2020). The very nature of nursing facilities (multiple residents staying in one room, staff attending to residents back to back) makes it an especially vulnerable environment for COVID-19 to spread.

Because of this, visiting is limited at the moment. The COVID-19 pandemic essentially takes the advice from this guide and puts it through a blender. It certainly makes it more difficult to stay involved when you're unable to be physically present.

While we may understand adjusting visitation for the safety of the at-risk SNF population, it is easy to see the downfalls of the lack of outside contact. In my experience, more residents are feeling aimless, depressed, and missing their loved ones than ever before. It is a completely disheartening time for them.

Still, we see supportive families bringing the supplies they always have, making phone and video calls on an even more regular basis, and visiting outside sliding doors and glass barriers to make the closest-to-physical-contact possible. This isn't a remedy to the isolation, but it certainly is a step in the right direction.

At the moment of writing this, nobody knows when visitation will become completely normal again. Whatever is coming up next in these unknown waters we're treading, the hope is that soon we will be able to return to the normalcy that we once knew.

In the meantime, do your best with what the situation entails. We would love to be able to follow every instruction in this guide to show our loved one the most support, but the current reality makes it difficult.

Do your best for your loved one, and your best will reflect on them.

CONCLUSION

This guide is a general overview of the questions I've heard from patients and their loved ones during my time working in a SNF. No doubt, you may have questions that are not answered in these pages; however, it is my sincerest hope that, more than anything, you have gathered an overall sense of understanding in being involved in your loved one's care. This knowledge and empowerment is truly the driving force in gaining the confidence to help your loved one with their care.

Here are a few takeaways I can provide you as you walk with your loved one on their SNF journey (or if you're on this journey yourself):

- **Treat your loved one's care staff with respect.** This is probably the largest point to drive home. Your kindness toward these extremely hard-working individuals will truly shape your loved one's experience— and yours. Establishing genuine relationships with your loved one's caregivers and giving them respect is the best advice I can give you on your journey of caring for your loved one in a SNF. While there may be instances when you need to trade in your kindness for firmness, an overall attitude of gratitude will take you much, much further in empowering your loved one on their SNF journey.
  Should your discussions with your loved one's caregivers not seem to take you anywhere, hopefully you now have a better understanding of the hierarchy of a SNF and where you can go to address your concerns.
- **Remember that a SNF is a healthcare facility.** Some facilities are residential in nature, meaning individuals live there, but it is a medical facility first and

foremost. Keep this in mind when it comes to everyday comforts, as they may not always be provided in the same ways we are used to at home.

As a healthcare facility, a SNF must operate under guidelines to ensure they are functioning safely. This means prohibiting certain items, imposing visitor hours, and making rules around things that can be brought in or taken out. Try to approach these regulations with an air of understanding that these guidelines need to be followed for them to operate lawfully.

- **Visiting makes a big difference.** Visiting at any capacity you can has, time and time again, proven to me to be a great indicator of success and quality of life in individuals I've cared for. While frequent visits may or may not be viable in your particular case, hopefully you have learned other ways of keeping involved and informed in your loved one's care.
- **If your loved one is staying long-term, bringing comforts from home helps.** I have truly noticed the difference decorating a room, bringing a favorite throw blanket, or providing familiar hobbies can have for a resident staying long-term in a SNF.
- **Take care of yourself and your well-being.** Understand that taking time for yourself is extremely important to avoid burnout. We can't care for and empower our loved ones if we are stressed beyond measure. Having a loved one in a nursing facility can be a challenge for both them as well as those providing support from the outside. In the case of a loved one who cannot speak for themselves, we may find ourselves having to be their voice time and time again.

Take time out for yourself and delegate responsibilities to others, if possible, to avoid being overwhelmed. Go easy on yourself: the fact you are reading this means you are already taking steps toward informing yourself how to best help your loved one!

If you've even browsed through some of this guide, you are taking steps in the right direction to helping your loved one prosper in a skilled nursing facility. Hopefully, with your efforts and the efforts of their facility, your loved one will feel cared for, cherished, and respected—just as they deserve.

CHECKLIST

Directions: Use this checklist as needed to ensure you have addressed some of the most important areas around your loved one's nursing facility stay. This may be especially helpful during the initial days and weeks.

The first few days:

- ☐ If my loved one is taking medication for symptoms (i.e., pain or nausea), have I made sure they were given a dose prior to leaving the hospital to ensure a smooth transition?
- ☐ Has my loved one arrived at the facility? What room is he/she in?
- ☐ Have I spoken to the nurse about any immediate concerns, if any?
- ☐ Have I compiled a list of questions to bring to the team during the initial care conference?
- ☐ Have I considered what items to bring my loved one to smooth their transition?
- ☐ Have I ensured anything I've brought my loved one is clearly labeled or will be labeled by the facility?
- ☐ Do I know some of the main departments I can speak with regarding questions?

Ongoing questions to consider, especially with longer stays:

- ☐ Have I shared my loved one's dietary preferences with the dietary staff? Am I able to safely bring some of their preferred foods?

- ☐ Have I ensured that the clothing I've brought is comfortable and easy to put on/takeoff?
- ☐ Did I make sure to bring comfortable shoes?
- ☐ Did I bring some of my loved one's preferred toiletries?
- ☐ Have I brought some of my loved one's comforts from home? A pillow or throw blanket? Some family photos? TV headphones? Earplugs? Cellphone?
- ☐ Have I brought organization bins for my loved one's things to maintain their belongings?
- ☐ Have I brought items to encourage memory? A visible clock? Calendar?
- ☐ How is my loved one getting along with their roommate(s)?
- ☐ Is my loved one getting out of bed? What equipment are they using (i.e., walker, cane, wheelchair)?
- ☐ If my loved one is spending most of their time in bed, are interventions in place to prevent them from getting pressure sores? If possible, are there interventions in place to help them out of bed more often?
- ☐ Does my loved one have things to keep them engaged throughout the day? Have I spoken with the activities staff about their leisure time?
- ☐ Is my loved one on therapy? If so, how is their progress?
- ☐ If my loved one isn't on therapy, are they receiving RNA or FMP services to maintain their function?
- ☐ How are my loved one's mental health and emotional state? Would they benefit from psychological services?
- ☐ Is my loved one receiving dental or vision services?
- ☐ If my loved one needs podiatry services, are they scheduled to see them?
- ☐ How does my loved one get to/from appointments?
- ☐ Do I know how who to speak to in case I notice a medical change in my loved one?

- [ ] Do I know who I can contact for complaints?
- [ ] Can I recognize some signs of elder abuse?
- [ ] Do I know who to contact in the case of suspected abuse or neglect?

Hopefully, this checklist does not seem daunting. All items may not apply to your loved one's specific case, especially if they are only staying for a short time. You can direct any questions you have to the appropriate staff; however, if you don't know who you need to speak with, feel comfortable asking!

RESOURCES

Suspected Abuse Reporting

Report a suspected case of abuse to Adult Protective Services (APS) by state:

State	Phone Number
Alabama	1-800-458-7214
Alaska	1-800-478-9996
Arizona	877-767-2385
Arkansas	800-482-8049
California	1-833-401-0832
Colorado	Number varies by county. Contact the general Department of Human Services line at 303-866-5700 to be provided the correct contact number.
Connecticut	1-888-385-4225
Delaware	1-800-223-9074
Florida	1-800-962-2873
Georgia	1-866-552-4464
Hawaii	808-832-5115

Idaho Eastern Idaho North Central Idaho Northern Idaho South Central Idaho Southeast Idaho Southwest Idaho	Numbers vary by region: 1-208-522-5391 1-208-743-5580 1-208-667-3179 1-208-736-2122 1-208-233-4032 1-208-898-7060
Illinois	1-866-800-1409
Indiana	800-992-6978
Iowa	1-800-362-2178
Kansas	1-800-922-5330
Kentucky	502-564-7043
Louisiana	1-800-898-4910
Maine	1-800-624-8404
Maryland	1-800-332-6347
Massachusetts	800-922-2275
Michigan	855-444-3911
Minnesota	1-844-880-1574
Mississippi	844-437-6282
Missouri	1-800-392-0210
Montana	1-844-277-9300
Nebraska	800-652-1999

Nevada Las Vegas/Clark County All Other Areas	Number varies by region: 702-486-6930 888-729-0571
New Hampshire	800-949-0470
New Jersey	609-588-6501
New Mexico	1-866-654-3219
New York	1-844-697-3505
North Carolina	Number varies by county. Contact the general Department of Health and Human Services office at 1-800-662-7030 to be provided the correct contact number.
North Dakota	1-855-462-5465
Ohio	855-644-6277 (855-OHIO-APS)
Oklahoma	1-800-522-3511
Oregon	1-855-503-SAFE (7233)
Pennsylvania	1-800-490-8505
Rhode Island	401-462-0555
South Carolina	1-888-227-3487 (1-888-CARE4US)
South Dakota	1-833-663-9673
Tennessee	1-888-277-8366
Texas	800-252-5400
Utah	1-800-371-7897
Vermont	800-564-1612

Virginia	888-832-3858
Washington	1-877-734-6277
West Virginia	1-800-352-6513
Wisconsin	Number varies by county. Contact the general Department of Health Services office at 608-261-8319 to be provided the correct contact number.
Wyoming	1-800-457-3659

Complaint Filing

File a complaint against a Medicare *provider* (not an institution): 1-800-MEDICARE (1-800-633-4227)

File a complaint about a *nursing home* with your state's appropriate surveying agency:

State	Number
Alabama	1-800-252-1818
Alaska	1-907-334-2483
Arizona	602-542-1000
Arkansas	1-800-482-8988
California	1-800-236-9747
Colorado	1-800 886-7689 Ext 2800
Connecticut	860-509-7400
Delaware	1-877-453-0012
District of Columbia	202-442-5833
Florida	1-888-419-3456
Georgia	404-657-2700
Hawaii	808-692-7420
Idaho	208-334-6626
Illinois	1-800-252-4343
Indiana	1-800-246-8909
Iowa	515-281-7102

Kansas	1-800-842-0078
Kentucky	Business Hours: 502-564-7963 Non-Business Hours: 1-800-372-2973
Louisiana	225-342-0138
Maine	207-287-3707
Maryland	1-877-402-8218
Massachusetts	617-753-8150
Michigan	1-800-882-6006
Minnesota	1-800-369-7994
Mississippi	601-576-7400
Missouri	1-800-392-0210
Montana	406-444-2099
Nebraska	402-471-0316
Nevada	Carson City 775-687-4475 Las Vegas 702-486-6515
New Hampshire	603-271-4592
New Jersey	1-800-367-6543
New Mexico	1-800-445-6242
New York	1-866-881-2809
North Carolina	1-800-624-3004
North Dakota	701-328-2352
Ohio	1-800-342-0553

Oklahoma	1-800-747-8419
Oregon	971-673-0540
Pennsylvania	1-800-222-0989
Rhode Island	401-222-5200
South Carolina	803-545-4370
South Dakota	1-800-738-2301
Tennessee	1-877-287-0010
Texas	1-888-973-0022
Utah	1-800-662-4157
Vermont	1-800-564-1612
Virginia	1-800-955-1819
Washington	1-800-562-6078
West Virginia	304-558-0050
Wisconsin	608-266-8481
Wyoming	1-800-548-1367

Advocacy Groups and Resources Aiding the Elderly

Administration on Aging (AoA) - principle agency of the U.S. Department of Health and Human Services aimed at fostering independence and well-being for older adults. Under the AoA are funding and the provision of adult health day cares, caregiving services, legal justice for elder abuse, behavioral health resources, and much more.
202-401-4634
https://acl.gov/contact

Alzheimer's Association - an organization aimed at providing support and care for those affected by Alzheimer's Disease as well as their loved ones. Local chapters provide face-to-face support groups and education, as well as online resources. A free national helpline is available 24/7 with qualified professionals.
800-272-3900
https://www.alz.org/

Eldercare Locator - a public service provided by the U.S. Administration on Aging (AoA) that provides access to local resources by simply inputting your location. The results can direct you to adult day health cares, local organizations for the elderly, healthcare insurance counseling, and much more.
1-800-677-1116
https://eldercare.acl.gov/

Legal Services Corporation (LSC) - a legal nonprofit organization that provides low-income Americans access to legal services and representation through a grants/selection process.
202-295-1500
https://www.lsc.gov/

National Center on Elder Abuse (NCEA) - an organization aimed at improving the national response to elder abuse by providing resources to professionals, advocates, and families alike. The NCEA is a part of the Administration on Aging (AoA).
1-855-500-3537
https://ncea.acl.gov/

The National Consumer Voice for Quality Long-Term Care - an organization that provides knowledge and resources to patients and families alike in advocating for needs in long-term care settings.
202-332-2275
info@theconsumervoice.org

The National Council on Aging (NCOA) - a society that provides organizations and individuals resources to help with the aging process. Signing up for their email updates can keep you up to date on advocacy efforts.
https://www.ncoa.org/page/contact-us

The Long Term Care Community Coalition (LTCCC) - organization aimed at improving the quality of care and quality of life of individuals living in long-term care, assisted living, and other residential settings.
212-385-0355
feedback@LTCCC.org

State Health Insurance Assistance Programs (SHIP) - Every state has a SHIP that provides one-on-one insurance counseling and assistance with Medicare needs and questions. Locate your SHIP online or by calling the national number.
877-839-2675
https://www.shiptacenter.org/

REFERENCES

Adult Protective Services. (2020). Department of Social Services. https://www.cdss.ca.gov/inforesources/adult-protective-services

Association of American Medical Colleges. (2021). *Specialty Profiles*. Careers in Medicine. https://www.aamc.org/cim/explore-options/specialty-profiles.

Bhattacharya, S., & Mishra, R. K. (2015). Pressure ulcers: Current understanding and newer modalities of treatment. *Indian Journal of Plastic Surgery*, 48(01), 004-016. doi:10.4103/0970-0358.155260

Center for Devices and Radiological Health. (2010, April). *A Guide to Bed Safety Bed Rails in Hospitals, Nursing Homes and Home Health Care: The Facts*. Retrieved December 19, 2020, from https://www.fda.gov/medical-devices/hospital-beds/guide-bed-safety-bed-rails-hospitals-nursing-homes-and-home-health-care-facts

Grabowski, D. C., & Mitchell, S. L. (2009). Family oversight and the quality of nursing home care for residents with advanced dementia [Abstract]. *Med Care*, 47(5), 568-74. doi:10.1097/MLR.0b013e318195fce7

Harrington, C., Dellefield, M., Halifax, E., Fleming, M., & Bakerjian, D. (2020, June 29). *Appropriate Nurse Staffing Levels for U.S. Nursing Homes*. Retrieved January 24, 2021, from https://www.ncbi.nlm.nih.gov/pmc/articles/PMC7328494/

Iinuma, T., Arai, Y., Abe, Y., Takayama, M., Fukumoto, M., Fukui, Y., . . . Komiyama, K. (2014). Denture Wearing during Sleep Doubles the Risk of Pneumonia in the Very Elderly. *Journal of Dental Research*, 94(3_suppl). doi:10.1177/0022034514552493

Lyder, C. H.,& Ayello, E. A. (2008). Pressure Ulcers: A Patient Safety Issue. In 923054224 724415729 R. Hughes (Author), Patient safety and quality: An evidence-based handbook for nurses (p. 269). Rockville, MD: Agency for Healthcare Research and Quality, U.S. Dept. of Health and Human Services.

National Council on Aging. (2021, February 23). *Get the Facts on Elder Abuse*. https://www.ncoa.org/public-policy-action/elder-justice/elder-abuse-facts/.

National Council on Aging. (2021). *Get the Facts on Falls Prevention*. https://www.ncoa.org/article/get-the-facts-on-falls-prevention.

Quagliarello, V., Ginter, S., Han, L., Ness, P. V., Allore, H., & Tinetti, M. (2005). Modifiable Risk Factors for Nursing Home-Acquired Pneumonia. *Clinical Infectious Diseases*, 40(1), 1-6. doi:10.1086/426023

U.S. Centers for Medicare & Medicaid Services. (2020, August 27). Federal Regulatory Groups for Long Term Care. CMS.gov. https://www.cms.gov/Medicare/Provider-Enrollment-and-Certification/GuidanceforLawsAndRegulations/Downloads/List-of-Revised-FTags.pdf.

U.S. Centers for Medicare & Medicaid Services. (n.d.). *Appendix PP - Guidance to Surveyors for Long Term Care Facilities*. CMS.gov. https://www.cms.gov/Regulations-and-Guidance/Guidance/Manuals/downloads/som107ap_pp_guidelines_ltcf.pdf.

U.S. Centers for Medicare & Medicaid Services. (n.d.). Skilled nursing facility (SNF) care. Medicare.gov. https://www.medicare.gov/coverage/skilled-nursing-facility-snf-care.

U.S. Centers for Medicare & Medicaid Services. (n.d.). *Skilled nursing facility rights*. Medicare.gov. https://www.medicare.gov/what-medicare-covers/what-part-a-covers/skilled-nursing-facility-rights.

Williamson, E., Walker, A. J., Bhaskaran, K. J., Bacon, S., Bates, C., Morton, C. E., . . .Goldacre, B. (2020). OpenSAFELY: Factors associated with COVID-19-related hospital death in the linked electronic health records of 17 million adult NHS patients. doi:10.1101/2020.05.06.20092999

www.ingramcontent.com/pod-product-compliance
Lightning Source LLC
Chambersburg PA
CBHW071415210526
45465CB00001B/393